# Vitamin K Levels in Common Foods

Timothy S. Harlan, M.D.
Dr. Gourmet
www.DrGourmet.com

# CONTENTS

About Coumadin (warfarin)                     1

Amounts of Vitamin K in Common Foods    13
Alphabetical List

Amounts of Vitamin K in Common Foods    66
By Amount, Descending

# ABOUT COUMADIN® (WARFARIN)

Coumadin® (warfarin) is a prescription medication used for anticoagulation. It is often referred to as "a blood thinner," but that is not really an accurate description. It works by inhibiting enzymes that lead to blood clotting. It is the only well researched, effective oral medication that for this purpose. (Other brand names for warfarin are Coumadin, Jantoven, Marevan, and Waran.)

Its primary use is to treat or prevent blood clots. When the blood clots in a vein or artery, physicians refer to it as a *thrombus*. When the thrombus breaks free and travels to other parts of the body it is known as an *embolus*. A common problem known as deep vein thrombosis (DVT) occurs when such clots form in the large veins in the legs or arms. These will commonly form and then break free and travel to the lungs, blocking blood flow, which is known as a pulmonary embolus (PE).

Other uses include:
> Pulmonary embolism
> Artificial heart valves
> Atrial fibrillation
> Atrial flutter
> Transient ischemic attacks (TIAs)
> Stroke
> Heart attack
> Blockages of the arteries
> After some surgeries

Those with disorders of the clotting system

I get the question all the time about how much Vitamin K is right for folks taking Coumadin® (warfarin). Unfortunately, there's no perfect study to guide just how much Vitamin K is too much for those taking Coumadin. Most physicians recommend limiting foods that contain very high or even moderate amounts of Vitamin K. At the same time there's never been a study to recommend severely limiting Vitamin K intake.

The Recommended Daily Allowance (RDA) for Vitamin K is 80 micrograms (mcg) for males and 70 mcg for females. Most ingredients contain small amounts -in the under 15 mcg range -so keeping an eye on foods that contain more than 20 -25 mcg per serving is a good rule of thumb.

Avoiding all Vitamin K might be just as much of a problem, however. Studies have clearly shown that eating foods that are higher in Vitamin K will have an effect on the effect of Coumadin and the INR. Most folks who either take warfarin or those who help patients manage their anti-coagulation know this but there is some research now that shows eating too little Vitamin K can have the same effect.

So what to do? How much is too much? How little is too little? It appears from what research we have that in those folks taking Coumadin 29 mcg was too little and 76 mcg just right to keep their INR stable.

While it's not a perfect way to look at the issue of how much is too much Vitamin K in the diet for warfarin users, another study showed an effect on the INR in those taking 150 -200 mcg per day in Vitamin K supplements. These are the levels found in Vitamin K rich foods such as spinach, collard greens and broccoli. For the number of folks who use this medication and the fact that there's no great replacement on the horizon, it is a shame that a large study has not been done to help answer this question more clearly. For the time being we have to be content with the small studies that point toward an optimum level that is near the RDA guidelines for Vitamin K.

## How it Works

Warfarin is a synthetic version of a class of chemicals known as coumarins. These are found in many plants, such as woodruff, lavender and licorice. It was named by combining the acronym for the Wisconsin Alumni Research Foundation (WARF) and the suffix for coumarin (arin). The Foundation provided the original research grants, and it was indeed originally developed as rat poison, but is seldom used as a rat poison today because similar but much more potent forms are now available for that purpose.

Warfarin's anticoagulant effect works because the drug inhibits production of proteins known as "clotting factors." These proteins are produced in the liver and are dependent on an adequate supply of Vitamin K. The clotting factor proteins are the foundation of the "intrinsic" clotting pathway. There are many proteins that work together, and warfarin blocks four of them: Factors VII, IX, X, and II. Creation of these proteins in the liver is dependent on Vitamin K, which can come from dietary sources but can also be created by bacteria in the large intestine. After being absorbed, Vitamin K is stored in the liver. Consequently Vitamin K is the vital regulatory step for the production of the clotting Factors VII, IX, X, and II.

Warfarin blocks the action of vitamin K within the liver by blocking the absorption sites in the liver needed for the uptake of vitamin K. With the lowered ability for Vitamin K absorption, there is reduced production of the clotting factors. Consequently, dietary intake of Vitamin K affects the effectiveness of warfarin.

## Prescribing Coumadin® (warfarin)

Doctors prescribe Coumadin to patients who are prone to thrombosis and also to prevent them in those who have already formed blood clots. There are numerous conditions that can lead to clot formation, including prosthetic heart valves, atrial fibrillation, deep venous thrombosis and pulmonary embolism. There are also those with inherited problems with clotting factors, like antiphospholipid syndrome and factor five leiden, for whom we prescribe warfarin to prevent clotting. Sometimes the drug is used after myocardial infarction (heart attack) and stroke.

Finding the correct dose of warfarin for patients is complicated by the fact that it interacts with many other over-the-counter and prescription medications, as well as supplements. This interaction can cause Coumadin to be more or less effective. The activity of the drug has to be monitored by frequent blood testing for the international normalized ratio (INR). If the INR is high, the dose is too high. Conversely, if the INR is too low, the medication dose needs to be increased. (We used to use a test, the Prothrombin Time, sometimes called the "Pro Time" or PT, but its accuracy varied between labs. Now results are standardized through the use of the INR.)

## Interactions

There are commonly used antibiotics such as erythromycin (Eryc), clarithromycin (Biaxin) and metronidazole (Flagyl) that can markedly increase the effect of Coumadin. In some cases, using antibiotics often changes the amount of the normal bacteria in the intestines and can alter the amount of Vitamin K absorbed into the body.

Genetics also play a factor in how warfarin is processed in the body. There are tests recently approved by the Food and Drug Administration that can help guide dosing of warfarin.

## Adjusting the Dose

It is very important that you always know when will be your next blood test for the INR. It is equally important to know what dose you are taking. It's a good idea to keep a warfarin calendar to help you keep track. Get a small calendar and carry it with you (in your wallet or purse). Write your doses of warfarin in the appropriate days until the next blood test. When you take your dose, circle that day so that you know you have taken it. In the day scheduled for your blood test, write "Get INR" to remind yourself. After the test, if you have not heard from your doctor's office about your results, call them for any new instructions.

The target level of the INR will depend on why you are taking warfarin. In most cases the target range for INR is 2.0-3.0. In some cases, however, the range is higher. Your doctor will set the target based on your particular condition.

Most physicians prefer for their patients to take warfarin in the evening. This is primarily because blood tests are typically taken in the morning, and it will give your doctor time to contact you after your INR is checked. He or she can then change the dose, if needed, before you take your evening medication. There are now home testing kits available and insurance companies are paying for these more and more. Check with your doctor and your insurance company to see if you qualify.

You **must** tell **any** doctor who prescribes medicine for you that you are taking warfarin. If you have any unusual bleeding let your doctor know right away. Call your doctor with any questions or issues earlier rather than later. It's a good idea to have a "Medic Alert" bracelet stating that you are taking warfarin.

## Common Side Effects

### Rash

On rare occasions warfarin can cause a generalized rash. This has a lacy red pattern and you should call your doctor immediately to discuss this.

### Bleeding

The most concerning side effect of warfarin is hemorrhage (bleeding). The risk of severe bleeding is small -on the order of 1 to 2%. In most cases where doctors prescribe warfarin, the benefit will far outweigh the risk. This is why it is so important to take care with your diet as well as other supplements that might interact with the drug.

It may seem difficult and irritating at times for your doctor to have you get your INR level checked, but this is what allows him or her to carefully regulate the drug and reduce the risk of bleeding.

### Warfarin necrosis

A rare complication of warfarin is can be necrosis, or death of skin tissues. This happens more often in people with a deficiency of protein C.

### Purple toe syndrome

Another rare side effect is known as purple toe syndrome. It generally occurs early after starting the medication --usually within 3 to 8 weeks. It is thought to be the result of small bits of cholesterol breaking loose from large arteries and flowing into the smaller blood vessels of the feet.

### Osteoporosis

Several studies have shown a link between warfarin use and osteoporosis related fractures.

# Contraindications

Pregnant women or women who can easily become pregnant should not take warfarin. This is especially true during the first trimester, as it is known to cause deformations of the face and bones. During the third trimester there is a high risk of bleeding. There are alternatives such as heparin, however.

# Other Interactions

Taking other medications can also increase the risk of bleeding. The most common are antiplatelet drugs such as aspirin, clopidogrel or nonsteroidal anti-inflammatory drugs like ibuprofen (Advil) or naproxyn (Aleve, Naprosyn).

There are many other drug-to-drug interactions, and because of genetic factors the body's processing of the drug can vary widely between patients.

Excessive alcohol use can also affect how warfarin is processed in the liver and elevate the INR. Most physicians will caution patients about the use of alcohol while taking warfarin. Commonly doctors will allow a few drinks after INR is stable.

Foods that are high in Vitamin K have also been reported to interact with warfarin.

## Supplements

Warfarin also interacts with many herbs, including (but not limited to):
Ginkgo Biloba
St. John's Wort
American Ginseng
Garlic as a supplement (not fresh garlic)

# AMOUNTS OF VITAMIN K
# IN COMMON FOODS
# ALPHABETICAL LIST

| Description | Common Measure | Mcg Vit. K |
|---|---|---|
| Alcoholic beverage, beer, light | 12 fl oz | 0.0 |
| Alcoholic beverage, beer, regular, all | 12 fl oz | 0.0 |
| Alcoholic beverage, daiquiri, prepared-from-recipe | 2 fl oz | 0.1 |
| Alcoholic beverage, distilled, all (gin, rum, vodka, whiskey) 80 proof | 1.5 fl oz | 0.0 |
| Alcoholic beverage, distilled, all (gin, rum, vodka, whiskey) 86 proof | 1.5 fl oz | 0.0 |
| Alcoholic beverage, distilled, all (gin, rum, vodka, whiskey) 90 proof | 1.5 fl oz | 0.0 |
| Alcoholic beverage, liqueur, coffee, 53 proof | 1.5 fl oz | 0.0 |
| Alcoholic beverage, pina colada, prepared-from-recipe | 4.5 fl oz | 0.1 |
| Alcoholic beverage, wine, dessert, dry | 3.5 fl oz | 0.0 |
| Alcoholic beverage, wine, dessert, sweet | 3.5 fl oz | 0.0 |

| | | |
|---|---|---|
| Alfalfa seeds, sprouted, raw | 1 cup | 10.1 |
| Apple juice, canned or bottled, unsweetened, without added ascorbic acid | 1 cup | 0.0 |
| Apples, dried, sulfured, uncooked | 5 rings | 1.0 |
| Apples, raw, with skin | 1 apple | 3.0 |
| Apples, raw, without skin | 1 cup | 0.7 |
| Applesauce, canned, sweetened, without salt | 1 cup | 1.5 |
| Applesauce, canned, unsweetened, without added ascorbic acid | 1 cup | 1.5 |
| Apricots, canned, heavy syrup pack, with skin, solids and liquids | 1 cup | 5.7 |
| Apricots, canned, juice pack, with skin, solids and liquids | 1 cup | 5.4 |
| Apricots, dried, sulfured, uncooked | 10 halves | 1.1 |
| Apricots, raw | 1 apricot | 1.2 |
| Artichokes, (globe or french), cooked, boiled, drained, without salt | 1 cup | 24.9 |
| Artichokes, (globe or french), cooked, boiled, drained, without salt | 1 medium | 17.8 |
| Asparagus, canned, drained solids | 4 spears | 29.7 |
| Asparagus, cooked, boiled, drained | 4 spears | 30.4 |
| Asparagus, frozen, cooked, boiled, drained, without salt | 4 spears | 48.0 |
| Asparagus, frozen, cooked, boiled, drained, without salt | 1 cup | 144.0 |

| | | |
|---|---|---|
| Avocados, raw, California | 1 oz | 6.0 |
| Bagels, cinnamon-raisin | 4" bagel | 0.6 |
| Bagels, cinnamon-raisin | 3-1/2" bagel | 0.5 |
| Bagels, plain, enriched, with calcium propionate (includes onion, poppy, sesame) | 4" bagel | 1.0 |
| Bagels, plain, enriched, with calcium propionate (includes onion, poppy, sesame) | 3-1/2" bagel | 0.8 |
| Baking chocolate, unsweetened, squares | 1 square | 2.7 |
| Bamboo shoots, canned, drained solids | 1 cup | 0.0 |
| Bananas, raw | 1 cup | 0.8 |
| Bananas, raw | 1 banana | 0.6 |
| Barley, pearled, cooked | 1 cup | 1.3 |
| Barley, pearled, raw | 1 cup | 4.4 |
| Beans, baked, canned, plain or vegetarian | 1 cup | 2.0 |
| Beans, baked, canned, with franks | 1 cup | 2.6 |
| Beans, baked, canned, with pork and sweet sauce | 1 cup | 2.0 |
| Beans, baked, canned, with pork and tomato sauce | 1 cup | 1.3 |
| Beans, kidney, red, mature seeds, canned | 1 cup | 5.6 |
| Beans, kidney, red, mature seeds, cooked, boiled, without salt | 1 cup | 5.8 |
| Beans, navy, mature seeds, cooked, boiled, without salt | 1 cup | 1.1 |
| Beans, pinto, mature seeds, cooked, boiled, without salt | 1 cup | 6.0 |

| | | |
|---|---|---|
| Beans, snap, green, canned, regular pack, drained solids | 1 cup | 13.4 |
| Beans, snap, green, cooked, boiled, drained, without salt | 1 cup | 20.0 |
| Beans, snap, green, frozen, cooked, boiled, drained without salt | 1 cup | 17.1 |
| Beans, snap, yellow, canned, regular pack, drained solids | 1 cup | 13.4 |
| Beans, snap, yellow, cooked, boiled, drained, without salt | 1 cup | 20.0 |
| Beans, snap, yellow, frozen, cooked, boiled, drained, without salt | 1 cup | 17.1 |
| Beef stew, canned entree | 1 cup | 8.1 |
| Beef, chuck, blade roast, separable lean only, trimmed to 1/4" fat, all grades, cooked, braised | 3 oz | 1.4 |
| Beef, cured, corned beef, canned | 3 oz | 1.4 |
| Beef, cured, dried | 1 oz | 0.0 |
| Beef, ground, 75% lean meat / 25% fat, patty, cooked, broiled | 3 oz | 1.9 |
| Beef, ground, 80% lean meat / 20% fat, patty, cooked, broiled | 3 oz | 1.4 |
| Beef, ground, 85% lean meat / 15% fat, patty, cooked, broiled | 3 oz | 1.0 |
| Beef, round, bottom round, separable lean and fat, trimmed to 1/8" fat, all grades, cooked, braised | 3 oz | 1.4 |
| Beef, round, bottom round, separable lean only, trimmed to 1/8" fat, all grades, cooked, braised | 3 oz | 1.4 |

| Food | Serving | Vitamin K |
|---|---|---|
| Beef, round, eye of round, separable lean and fat, trimmed to 1/8" fat, all grades, cooked, roasted | 3 oz | 1.2 |
| Beef, round, eye of round, separable lean only, trimmed to 1/8" fat, all grades, cooked, roasted | 3 oz | 1.6 |
| Beef, top sirloin, separable lean and fat, trimmed to 1/8" fat, all grades, cooked, broiled | 3 oz | 1.4 |
| Beef, top sirloin, separable lean only, trimmed to 1/8" fat, all grades, cooked, broiled | 3 oz | 1.2 |
| Beef, variety meats and by-products, liver, cooked, pan-fried | 3 oz | 3.3 |
| Beet greens, cooked, boiled, drained, without salt | 1 cup | 697.0 |
| Beets, canned, drained solids | 1 cup | 0.3 |
| Beets, canned, drained solids | 1 beet | 0.0 |
| Beets, cooked, boiled, drained | 1 beet | 0.1 |
| Beets, cooked, boiled, drained | 1 cup | 0.3 |
| Biscuits, plain or buttermilk, refrigerated dough, higher fat, baked | 2-1/2" biscuit | 0.6 |
| Biscuits, plain or buttermilk, refrigerated dough, lower fat, baked | 2-1/4" biscuit | 0.5 |
| Blackberries, raw | 1 cup | 28.5 |
| Blueberries, frozen, sweetened | 1 cup | 40.7 |
| Blueberries, raw | 1 cup | 28.0 |
| Bologna, beef and pork | 2 slices | 0.2 |
| Braunschweiger (a liver | 2 slices | 0.9 |

| | | |
|---|---|---|
| sausage), pork | | |
| Bread crumbs, dry, grated, plain | 1 oz | 1.9 |
| Bread crumbs, dry, grated, seasoned | 1 cup | 55.2 |
| Bread stuffing, bread, dry mix, prepared | 1/2 cup | 13.7 |
| Bread, egg | 1/2" slice | 0.4 |
| Bread, french or vienna (includes sourdough) | 1/2" slice | 0.3 |
| Bread, Indian, fry, made with lard (Navajo) | 10-1/2" bread | 1.3 |
| Bread, Indian, fry, made with lard (Navajo) | 5" bread | 0.7 |
| Bread, italian | 1 slice | 0.2 |
| Bread, mixed-grain (includes whole-grain, 7-grain) | 1 slice | 0.6 |
| Bread, mixed-grain, toasted (includes whole-grain, 7grain) | 1 slice | 0.5 |
| Bread, oatmeal | 1 slice | 0.4 |
| Bread, oatmeal, toasted | 1 slice | 0.4 |
| Bread, pita, white, enriched | 6-1/2" pita | 0.1 |
| Bread, pita, white, enriched | 4" pita | 0.1 |
| Bread, pumpernickel | 1 slice | 0.3 |
| Bread, pumpernickel, toasted | 1 slice | 0.3 |
| Bread, raisin, enriched | 1 slice | 0.4 |
| Bread, raisin, toasted, enriched | 1 slice | 0.5 |
| Bread, reduced-calorie, rye | 1 slice | 0.1 |
| Bread, reduced-calorie, wheat | 1 slice | 0.0 |
| Bread, reduced-calorie, white | 1 slice | 0.1 |
| Bread, rye | 1 slice | 0.4 |
| Bread, rye, toasted | 1 slice | 0.3 |
| Bread, wheat (includes wheat | 1 slice | 0.4 |

| | | |
|---|---|---|
| berry) | | |
| Bread, wheat, toasted (includes wheat berry) | 1 slice | 0.4 |
| Bread, white, commercially prepared (includes soft bread crumbs) | 1 cup | 1.4 |
| Bread, white, commercially prepared (includes soft bread crumbs) | 1 slice | 0.8 |
| Bread, white, commercially prepared, toasted | 1 slice | 0.7 |
| Bread, whole-wheat, commercially prepared | 1 slice | 0.6 |
| Bread, whole-wheat, commercially prepared, toasted | 1 slice | 0.6 |
| Broccoli, cooked, boiled, drained, without salt | 1 spear | 52.2 |
| Broccoli, cooked, boiled, drained, without salt | 1 cup | 220.1 |
| Broccoli, frozen, chopped, cooked, boiled, drained, without salt | 1 cup | 183.1 |
| Broccoli, raw | 1 spear | 31.5 |
| Broccoli, raw | 1 cup | 89.4 |
| Brussels sprouts, cooked, boiled, drained, without salt | 1 cup | 218.9 |
| Brussels sprouts, frozen, cooked, boiled, drained, without salt | 1 cup | 299.9 |
| Buckwheat flour, whole-groat | 1 cup | 8.4 |
| Buckwheat groats, roasted, cooked | 1 cup | 3.2 |
| Bulgur, cooked | 1 cup | 0.9 |
| Bulgur, dry | 1 cup | 2.7 |

| | | |
|---|---|---|
| Butter, salted | 1 tbsp | 1.0 |
| Butter, without salt | 1 tbsp | 1.0 |
| Cabbage, chinese (pak-choi), cooked, boiled, drained, without salt | 1 cup | 57.8 |
| Cabbage, cooked, boiled, drained, without salt | 1 cup | 73.4 |
| Cabbage, raw | 1 cup | 42.0 |
| Cabbage, red, raw | 1 cup | 26.7 |
| Cabbage, savoy, raw | 1 cup | 48.2 |
| Cake, angelfood, dry mix, prepared | 1 piece | 0.1 |
| Cake, boston cream pie, commercially prepared | 1 piece | 2.9 |
| Cake, fruitcake, commercially prepared | 1 piece | 0.6 |
| Cake, pound, commercially prepared, fat-free | 1 slice | 0.0 |
| Cake, snack cakes, creme-filled, chocolate with frosting | 1 cupcake | 1.4 |
| Cake, snack cakes, creme-filled, sponge | 1 cake | 0.6 |
| Cake, sponge, commercially prepared | 1 shortcake | 0.1 |
| Cake, white, prepared from recipe with coconut frosting | 1 piece | 4.6 |
| Cake, white, prepared from recipe without frosting | 1 piece | 3.8 |
| Candies, caramels | 1 piece | 0.2 |
| Candies, caramels, chocolate-flavor roll | 1 piece | 0.7 |
| Candies, carob | 1 oz | 2.2 |
| Candies, fudge, chocolate, prepared-from-recipe | 1 piece | 0.2 |
| Candies, fudge, chocolate, | 1 piece | 0.3 |

| | | |
|---|---|---|
| with nuts, prepared-fromrecipe | | |
| Candies, fudge, vanilla with nuts | 1 piece | 0.1 |
| Candies, fudge, vanilla, prepared-from-recipe | 1 piece | 0.1 |
| Candies, gumdrops, starch jelly pieces | 10 bears | 0.0 |
| Candies, gumdrops, starch jelly pieces | 1 medium | 0.0 |
| Candies, gumdrops, starch jelly pieces | 10 worms | 0.0 |
| Candies, hard | 1 small piece | 0.0 |
| Candies, hard | 1 piece | 0.0 |
| Candies, jellybeans | 10 large | 0.0 |
| Candies, KIT KAT Wafer Bar | 1 bar (1.5 oz) | 2.2 |
| Candies, M&M MARS, "M&M's" Milk Chocolate Candies | 10 pieces | 0.2 |
| Candies, M&M MARS, "M&M's" Peanut Chocolate Candies | 10 pieces | 0.6 |
| Candies, M&M MARS, MARS MILKY WAY Bar | 1 bar (2.15 oz) | 2.3 |
| Candies, M&M MARS, MARS MILKY WAY Bar | 1 fun size bar | 0.7 |
| Candies, M&M MARS, SNICKERS Bar | 1 bar (2 oz) | 1.1 |
| Candies, M&M MARS, STARBURST Fruit Chews | 1 piece | 0.1 |
| Candies, marshmallows | 1 cup | 0.0 |
| Candies, milk chocolate | 1 bar (1.55 oz) | 2.5 |
| Candies, milk chocolate | 10 pieces | 1.6 |

| | | |
|---|---|---|
| coated peanuts | | |
| Candies, milk chocolate coated raisins | 10 pieces | 0.4 |
| Candies, milk chocolate, with almonds | 1 bar (1.45 oz) | 2.1 |
| Candies, MR. GOODBAR Chocolate Bar | 1 bar (1.75 oz) | 1.8 |
| Candies, NESTLE, BUTTERFINGER Bar | 1 fun size bar | 0.1 |
| Candies, REESE'S Peanut Butter Cups | 1 package (contains 2) | 2.3 |
| Candies, semisweet chocolate | 1 cup | 9.4 |
| Candies, white chocolate | 1 cup | 15.5 |
| Carambola, (starfruit), raw | 1 cup | 0.0 |
| Carambola, (starfruit), raw | 1 fruit | 0.0 |
| Carbonated beverage, club soda | 12 fl oz | 0.0 |
| Carbonated beverage, cola, contains caffeine | 12 fl oz | 0.0 |
| Carbonated beverage, ginger ale | 12 fl oz | 0.0 |
| Carbonated beverage, low calorie, cola or pepper-type, with aspartame, contains caffeine | 12 fl oz | 0.0 |
| Carbonated beverage, low calorie, other than cola or pepper, without caffeine | 12 fl oz | 0.0 |
| Carbonated beverage, root beer | 12 fl oz | 0.0 |
| Carbonated beverage, SPRITE, lemon-lime, without caffeine | 12 fl oz | 0.0 |

| | | |
|---|---|---|
| Carob flour | 1 tbsp | 0.0 |
| Carrot juice, canned | 1 cup | 36.6 |
| Carrots, baby, raw | 1 medium | 0.9 |
| Carrots, canned, regular pack, drained solids | 1 cup | 14.3 |
| Carrots, cooked, boiled, drained, without salt | 1 cup | 21.4 |
| Carrots, frozen, cooked, boiled, drained, without salt | 1 cup | 19.9 |
| Carrots, raw | 1 carrot | 9.5 |
| Carrots, raw | 1 cup | 14.5 |
| Catsup | 1 tbsp | 0.4 |
| Catsup | 1 packet | 0.2 |
| Cauliflower, cooked, boiled, drained, without salt | 3 flowerets | 7.5 |
| Cauliflower, cooked, boiled, drained, without salt | 1 cup | 17.1 |
| Cauliflower, frozen, cooked, boiled, drained, without salt | 1 cup | 21.4 |
| Cauliflower, raw | 1 floweret | 2.1 |
| Cauliflower, raw | 1 cup | 16.0 |
| Celery, cooked, boiled, drained, without salt | 1 cup | 56.7 |
| Celery, cooked, boiled, drained, without salt | 1 stalk | 14.2 |
| Celery, raw | 1 stalk | 11.7 |
| Celery, raw | 1 cup | 35.2 |
| Cereals ready-to-eat, GENERAL MILLS, APPLE CINNAMON CHEERIOS | 3/4 cup | 0.5 |
| Cereals ready-to-eat, GENERAL MILLS, BASIC 4 | 1 cup | 1.5 |
| Cereals ready-to-eat, GENERAL MILLS, BERRY | 3/4 cup | 0.4 |

| | | |
|---|---|---|
| BERRY KIX | | |
| Cereals ready-to-eat, GENERAL MILLS, CHEERIOS | 1 cup | 0.5 |
| Cereals ready-to-eat, GENERAL MILLS, CINNAMON TOAST CRUNCH | 3/4 cup | 1.9 |
| Cereals ready-to-eat, GENERAL MILLS, COCOA PUFFS | 1 cup | 0.2 |
| Cereals ready-to-eat, GENERAL MILLS, Corn CHEX | 1 cup | 0.1 |
| Cereals ready-to-eat, GENERAL MILLS, GOLDEN GRAHAMS | 3/4 cup | 0.3 |
| Cereals ready-to-eat, GENERAL MILLS, HONEY NUT CHEERIOS | 1 cup | 0.5 |
| Cereals ready-to-eat, GENERAL MILLS, Honey Nut CHEX | 3/4 cup | 0.0 |
| Cereals ready-to-eat, GENERAL MILLS, HONEY NUT CLUSTERS | 1 cup | 0.4 |
| Cereals ready-to-eat, GENERAL MILLS, KIX | 1-1/3 cup | 0.2 |
| Cereals ready-to-eat, GENERAL MILLS, LUCKY CHARMS | 1 cup | 0.4 |
| Cereals ready-to-eat, GENERAL MILLS, RAISIN NUT BRAN | 1 cup | 1.2 |
| Cereals ready-to-eat, GENERAL MILLS, REESE'S PUFFS | 3/4 cup | 0.3 |
| Cereals ready-to-eat, GENERAL MILLS, Rice CHEX | 1-1/4 cup | 0.0 |

| | | |
|---|---|---|
| Cereals ready-to-eat, GENERAL MILLS, TOTAL Corn Flakes | 1-1/3 cup | 0.1 |
| Cereals ready-to-eat, GENERAL MILLS, TOTAL Raisin Bran | 1 cup | 0.9 |
| Cereals ready-to-eat, GENERAL MILLS, TRIX | 1 cup | 0.3 |
| Cereals ready-to-eat, GENERAL MILLS, Wheat CHEX | 1 cup | 0.4 |
| Cereals ready-to-eat, GENERAL MILLS, WHEATIES | 1 cup | 0.5 |
| Cereals ready-to-eat, GENERAL MILLS, Whole Grain TOTAL | 3/4 cup | 0.2 |
| Cereals ready-to-eat, KELLOGG, KELLOGG'S ALL-BRAN Original | 1/2 cup | 1.6 |
| Cereals ready-to-eat, KELLOGG, KELLOGG'S APPLE JACKS | 1 cup | 0.3 |
| Cereals ready-to-eat, KELLOGG, KELLOGG'S COCOA KRISPIES | 3/4 cup | 0.0 |
| Cereals ready-to-eat, KELLOGG, KELLOGG'S Complete Wheat Bran Flakes | 3/4 cup | 0.5 |
| Cereals ready-to-eat, KELLOGG, KELLOGG'S Corn Flakes | 1 cup | 0.0 |
| Cereals ready-to-eat, KELLOGG, KELLOGG'S CORN POPS | 1 cup | 0.0 |
| Cereals ready-to-eat, KELLOGG, KELLOGG'S | 1 cup | 0.0 |

| | | |
|---|---|---|
| CRISPIX | | |
| Cereals ready-to-eat, KELLOGG, KELLOGG'S FROOT LOOPS | 1 cup | 0.1 |
| Cereals ready-to-eat, KELLOGG, KELLOGG'S FROSTED FLAKES | 3/4 cup | 0.1 |
| Cereals ready-to-eat, KELLOGG, KELLOGG'S FROSTED MINI WHEATS, bite size | 1 cup | 0.8 |
| Cereals ready-to-eat, KELLOGG, KELLOGG'S PRODUCT 19 | 1 cup | 0.2 |
| Cereals ready-to-eat, KELLOGG, KELLOGG'S RAISIN BRAN | 1 cup | 1.0 |
| Cereals ready-to-eat, KELLOGG, KELLOGG'S RICE KRISPIES | 1-1/4 cup | 0.0 |
| Cereals ready-to-eat, KELLOGG, KELLOGG'S RICE KRISPIES TREATS Cereal | 3/4 cup | 0.3 |
| Cereals ready-to-eat, KELLOGG, KELLOGG'S SMACKS | 3/4 cup | 0.3 |
| Cereals ready-to-eat, KELLOGG, KELLOGG'S SPECIAL K | 1 cup | 0.2 |
| Cereals ready-to-eat, KELLOGG'S FROSTED MINI-WHEATS, original | 1 cup | 0.8 |
| Cereals ready-to-eat, QUAKER, CAP'N CRUNCH | 3/4 cup | 0.4 |
| Cereals ready-to-eat, QUAKER, CAP'N CRUNCH | 3/4 cup | 0.4 |

| | | |
|---|---|---|
| with CRUNCHBERRIES | | |
| Cereals ready-to-eat, QUAKER, CAP'N CRUNCH'S PEANUT BUTTER CRUNCH | 3/4 cup | 0.3 |
| Cereals ready-to-eat, QUAKER, Honey Nut Heaven | 1 cup | 0.6 |
| Cereals ready-to-eat, QUAKER, Low Fat 100% Natural Granola with Raisins | 1/2 cup | 1.5 |
| Cereals ready-to-eat, QUAKER, QUAKER 100% Natural Cereal with oats, honey, and raisins | 1/2 cup | 2.1 |
| Cereals ready-to-eat, QUAKER, QUAKER OAT LIFE, plain | 3/4 cup | 0.5 |
| Cereals ready-to-eat, wheat germ, toasted, plain | 1 tbsp | 0.3 |
| Cereals ready-to-eat, wheat, shredded, plain, sugar and salt free | 2 biscuits | 0.6 |
| Cereals, corn grits, white, regular and quick, enriched, cooked with water, without salt | 1 cup | 0.0 |
| Cereals, corn grits, yellow, regular and quick, enriched, cooked with water, without salt | 1 cup | 0.0 |
| Cereals, CREAM OF WHEAT, regular, cooked with water, without salt | 1 cup | 0.3 |
| Cereals, oats, instant, fortified, plain, prepared with water | 1 packet | 0.9 |
| Cereals, oats, regular and quick and instant, unenriched, cooked with water, without salt | 1 cup | 7.5 |
| Cereals, QUAKER, Instant | 1 packet | 0.8 |

| | | |
|---|---|---|
| Oatmeal, maple and brown sugar, prepared with boiling water | | |
| Cereals, QUAKER,Instant Oatmeal, apples and cinnamon, prepared with boiling water | 1 packet | 0.7 |
| Cheese food, pasteurized process, american, without di sodium phosphate | 1 oz | 1.0 |
| Cheese spread, pasteurized process, american, without di sodium phosphate | 1 oz | 0.5 |
| Cheese, blue | 1 oz | 0.7 |
| Cheese, camembert | 1 wedge | 0.8 |
| Cheese, cheddar | 1 oz | 0.8 |
| Cheese, cottage, creamed, large or small curd | 1 cup | 0.8 |
| Cheese, cottage, creamed, with fruit | 1 cup | 0.9 |
| Cheese, cottage, lowfat, 1% milkfat | 1 cup | 0.2 |
| Cheese, cottage, lowfat, 2% milkfat | 1 cup | 0.5 |
| Cheese, cottage, nonfat, uncreamed, dry, large or small curd | 1 cup | 0.0 |
| Cheese, cream | 1 tbsp | 0.4 |
| Cheese, cream, fat free | 1 tbsp | 0.0 |
| Cheese, feta | 1 oz | 0.5 |
| Cheese, low fat, cheddar or colby | 1 oz | 0.2 |
| Cheese, mozzarella, part skim milk, low moisture | 1 oz | 0.4 |
| Cheese, mozzarella, whole | 1 oz | 0.7 |

| milk | | |
|---|---|---|
| Cheese, muenster | 1 oz | 0.7 |
| Cheese, parmesan, grated | 1 tbsp | 0.1 |
| Cheese, pasteurized process, american, with di sodium phosphate | 1 oz | 0.8 |
| Cheese, pasteurized process, swiss, with di sodium phosphate | 1 oz | 0.6 |
| Cheese, provolone | 1 oz | 0.6 |
| Cheese, ricotta, part skim milk | 1 cup | 1.7 |
| Cheese, ricotta, whole milk | 1 cup | 2.7 |
| Cheese, swiss | 1 oz | 0.7 |
| Cherries, sour, red, canned, water pack, solids and liquids (includes USDA commodity red tart cherries, canned) | 1 cup | 3.4 |
| Cherries, sweet, raw | 10 cherries | 1.4 |
| Chicken roll, light meat | 2 slices | 0.3 |
| Chicken, broilers or fryers, breast, meat and skin, cooked, fried, batter | 1/2 breast | 3.4 |
| Chicken, broilers or fryers, breast, meat only, cooked, roasted | 1/2 breast | 0.3 |
| Chicken, broilers or fryers, drumstick, meat only, cooked, roasted | 1 drumstick | 1.5 |
| Chicken, broilers or fryers, giblets, cooked, simmered | 1 cup | 0.0 |
| Chicken, broilers or fryers, thigh, meat only, cooked, roasted | 1 thigh | 2.0 |
| Chicken, canned, meat only, | 5 oz | 2.6 |

| | | |
|---|---|---|
| with broth | | |
| Chicken, liver, all classes, cooked, simmered | 1 liver | 0.0 |
| Chicken, stewing, meat only, cooked, stewed | 1 cup | 4.3 |
| Chickpeas (garbanzo beans, bengal gram), mature seeds, cooked, boiled, without salt | 1 cup | 6.6 |
| Chives, raw | 1 tbsp | 6.4 |
| Chocolate syrup | 1 tbsp | 0.1 |
| Chocolate-flavor beverage mix for milk, powder, without added nutrients | 2-3 heaping tsp | 2.1 |
| Chocolate-flavor beverage mix, powder, prepared with whole milk | 1 cup | 0.8 |
| Cocoa mix, no sugar added, powder | 1/2 oz envelope | 0.1 |
| Cocoa mix, powder | 3 heaping tsp | 0.3 |
| Cocoa mix, powder, prepared with water | 1 serving | 0.2 |
| Cocoa mix, with aspartame, powder, prepared from item 14196 | 1 serving | 1.3 |
| Cocoa, dry powder, unsweetened | 1 tbsp | 0.1 |
| Coffee, brewed from grounds, prepared with tap water | 6 fl oz | 0.2 |
| Coffee, brewed, espresso, restaurant-prepared | 2 fl oz | 0.1 |
| Coffee, instant, regular, prepared with water | 6 fl oz | 0.0 |
| Collards, cooked, boiled, | 1 cup | 836.0 |

| | | |
|---|---|---|
| drained, without salt | | |
| Collards, frozen, chopped, cooked, boiled, drained, without salt | 1 cup | 1059.4 |
| Cookies, brownies, commercially prepared | 1 brownie | 3.6 |
| Cookies, brownies, dry mix, special dietary, prepared | 1 brownie | 0.0 |
| Cookies, butter, commercially prepared, enriched | 1 cookie | 0.1 |
| Cookies, chocolate chip, commercially prepared, reg, higher fat, enriched | 1 cookie | 1.1 |
| Cookies, chocolate sandwich, with creme filling, regular | 1 cookie | 2.9 |
| Cookies, fig bars | 1 cookie | 0.9 |
| Cookies, graham crackers, plain or honey (includes cinnamon) | 2 squares | 0.6 |
| Cookies, graham crackers, plain or honey (includes cinnamon) | 1 cup | 3.9 |
| Cookies, molasses | 1 cookie, large (3-1/2" to 4" | 1.8 |
| Cookies, molasses | 1 cookie, medium | 0.8 |
| Cookies, oatmeal, commercially prepared, fat-free | 1 cookie | 0.1 |
| Cookies, oatmeal, commercially prepared, regular | 1 cookie | 2.0 |
| Cookies, peanut butter, commercially prepared, regular | 1 cookie | 0.7 |

| | | |
|---|---|---|
| Cookies, shortbread, commercially prepared, plain | 1 cookie | 0.8 |
| Cookies, sugar, commercially prepared, regular (includes vanilla) | 1 cookie | 1.3 |
| Cookies, sugar, prepared from recipe, made with margarine | 1 cookie | 3.6 |
| Cookies, sugar, refrigerated dough, baked | 1 cookie | 1.5 |
| Cookies, vanilla sandwich with creme filling | 1 cookie | 0.5 |
| Cookies, vanilla sandwich with creme filling | 1 cookie | 0.8 |
| Cookies, vanilla wafers, lower fat | 1 cookie | 0.2 |
| Corn, sweet, white, cooked, boiled, drained, without salt | 1 ear | 0.3 |
| Corn, sweet, yellow, canned, cream style, regular pack | 1 cup | 0.0 |
| Corn, sweet, yellow, canned, vacuum pack, regular pack | 1 cup | 0.0 |
| Corn, sweet, yellow, cooked, boiled, drained, without salt | 1 ear | 0.3 |
| Corn, sweet, yellow, frozen, kernels cut off cob, boiled, drained, without salt | 1 cup | 0.5 |
| Corn, sweet, yellow, frozen, kernels on cob, cooked, boiled, drained, without salt | 1 ear | 0.3 |
| Cornmeal, degermed, enriched, yellow | 1 cup | 0.4 |
| Cornmeal, whole-grain, yellow | 1 cup | 0.4 |
| Cornstarch | 1 tbsp | 0.0 |
| Couscous, cooked | 1 cup | 0.2 |
| Cowpeas (Blackeyes), | 1 cup | 43.9 |

| | | |
|---|---|---|
| immature seeds, cooked, boiled, drained, without salt | | |
| Cowpeas (blackeyes), immature seeds, frozen, cooked, boiled, drained, without salt | 1 cup | 62.6 |
| Cowpeas, common (blackeyes, crowder, southern), mature seeds, cooked, boiled, without salt | 1 cup | 2.9 |
| Crackers, cheese, regular | 10 crackers | 0.1 |
| Crackers, cheese, sandwich-type with peanut butter filling | 1 sandwich | 0.8 |
| Crackers, matzo, plain | 1 matzo | 0.1 |
| Crackers, melba toast, plain | 4 pieces | 0.2 |
| Crackers, rye, wafers, plain | 1 wafer | 0.6 |
| Crackers, saltines (includes oyster, soda, soup) | 4 crackers | 1.0 |
| Crackers, standard snack-type, regular | 4 crackers | 0.8 |
| Crackers, standard snack-type, sandwich, with cheese filling | 1 sandwich | 0.6 |
| Crackers, wheat, regular | 4 crackers | 0.8 |
| Crackers, whole-wheat | 4 crackers | 1.3 |
| Cranberry juice cocktail, bottled | 8 fl oz | 2.5 |
| Cranberry sauce, canned, sweetened | 1 slice | 0.8 |
| Cream substitute, liquid, with hydrogenated vegetable oil and soy protein | 1 tbsp | 0.4 |

| | | |
|---|---|---|
| Cream substitute, powdered | 1 tsp | 0.2 |
| Cream, fluid, half and half | 1 tbsp | 0.2 |
| Cream, fluid, heavy whipping | 1 tbsp | 0.5 |
| Cream, fluid, light (coffee cream or table cream) | 1 tbsp | 0.3 |
| Cream, fluid, light whipping | 1 tbsp | 0.4 |
| Cream, sour, cultured | 1 tbsp | 0.1 |
| Cream, sour, reduced fat, cultured | 1 tbsp | 0.1 |
| Cream, whipped, cream topping, pressurized | 1 tbsp | 0.1 |
| Croissants, butter | 1 croissant | 1.0 |
| Croutons, seasoned | 1 cup | 3.0 |
| Crustaceans, crab, alaska king, imitation, made from surimi | 3 oz | 0.1 |
| Crustaceans, crab, blue, canned | 1 cup | 0.1 |
| Crustaceans, crab, blue, cooked, moist heat | 3 oz | 0.1 |
| Crustaceans, lobster, northern, cooked, moist heat | 3 oz | 0.1 |
| Crustaceans, shrimp, mixed species, canned | 3 oz | 0.0 |
| Cucumber, peeled, raw | 1 cup | 8.6 |
| Cucumber, peeled, raw | 1 large | 20.2 |
| Cucumber, with peel, raw | 1 large | 49.4 |
| Cucumber, with peel, raw | 1 cup | 17.1 |
| Dandelion greens, cooked, boiled, drained, without salt | 1 cup | 203.6 |
| Danish pastry, cheese | 1 danish | 5.3 |
| Danish pastry, fruit, enriched (includes apple, cinnamon, raisin, lemon, raspberry, | 1 danish | 3.8 |

| | | |
|---|---|---|
| strawberry) | | |
| Dates, deglet noor | 5 dates | 1.1 |
| Dates, deglet noor | 1 cup | 4.8 |
| Dessert topping, powdered, 1.5 ounce prepared with 1/2 cup milk | 1 tbsp | 0.1 |
| Dessert topping, pressurized | 1 tbsp | 0.2 |
| Dessert topping, semi solid, frozen | 1 tbsp | 0.3 |
| Doughnuts, cake-type, plain (includes unsugared, old-fashioned) | 1 medium | 2.5 |
| Doughnuts, cake-type, plain (includes unsugared, old-fashioned) | 1 hole | 0.8 |
| Doughnuts, yeast-leavened, glazed, enriched (includes honey buns) | 1 medium | 5.8 |
| Doughnuts, yeast-leavened, glazed, enriched (includes honey buns) | 1 hole | 1.2 |
| Duck, domesticated, meat only, cooked, roasted | 1/2 duck | 8.4 |
| Eclairs, custard-filled with chocolate glaze, prepared from recipe | 1 eclair | 17.5 |
| Egg substitute, liquid | 1/4 cup | 0.5 |
| Egg, white, raw, fresh | 1 large | 0.0 |
| Egg, whole, cooked, fried | 1 large | 2.6 |
| Egg, whole, cooked, hard-boiled | 1 large | 0.2 |
| Egg, whole, cooked, poached | 1 large | 0.2 |
| Egg, whole, cooked, scrambled | 1 large | 2.4 |
| Egg, whole, raw, fresh | 1 extra | 0.2 |

| | large | |
|---|---|---|
| Egg, whole, raw, fresh | 1 large | 0.2 |
| Egg, whole, raw, fresh | 1 medium | 0.1 |
| Egg, yolk, raw, fresh | 1 large | 0.1 |
| Eggnog | 1 cup | 0.5 |
| Eggplant, cooked, boiled, drained, without salt | 1 cup | 2.9 |
| Endive, raw | 1 cup | 115.5 |
| English muffins, plain, enriched, with ca prop (includes sourdough) | 1 muffin | 0.7 |
| English muffins, plain, toasted, enriched, with calcium propionate (includes sourdough) | 1 muffin | 0.7 |
| Fast Food, Pizza Chain, 14" pizza, pepperoni topping, regular crust | 1 slice | 6.8 |
| Fast Foods, biscuit, with egg and sausage | 1 biscuit | 15.5 |
| Fast foods, chicken, breaded and fried, boneless pieces, plain | 6 pieces | 7.4 |
| Fast foods, chili con carne | 1 cup | 5.1 |
| Fast foods, coleslaw | 3/4 cup | 56.4 |
| Fast foods, french toast sticks | 5 sticks | 10.6 |
| Fast foods, ice milk, vanilla, soft-serve, with cone | 1 cone | 0.7 |
| Fast foods, potato, french fried in vegetable oil | 1 medium | 15.0 |
| Fast foods, potato, french fried in vegetable oil | 1 large | 18.9 |
| Fast foods, potato, french fried in vegetable oil | 1 small | 9.5 |

| | | |
|---|---|---|
| Figs, dried, uncooked | 2 figs | 5.9 |
| Fish, cod, Atlantic, canned, solids and liquid | 3 oz | 0.1 |
| Fish, fish portions and sticks, frozen, preheated | 1 portion (4" x 2" x 1/2") | 6.1 |
| Fish, fish portions and sticks, frozen, preheated | 1 stick (4" x 1" x 1/2") | 3.0 |
| Fish, flatfish (flounder and sole species), cooked, dry heat | 1 fillet | 0.1 |
| Fish, flatfish (flounder and sole species), cooked, dry heat | 3 oz | 0.1 |
| Fish, herring, Atlantic, pickled | 3 oz | 0.2 |
| Fish, pollock, walleye, cooked, dry heat | 1 fillet | 0.1 |
| Fish, pollock, walleye, cooked, dry heat | 3 oz | 0.1 |
| Fish, rockfish, Pacific, mixed species, cooked, dry heat | 1 fillet | 0.1 |
| Fish, rockfish, Pacific, mixed species, cooked, dry heat | 3 oz | 0.1 |
| Fish, roughy, orange, cooked, dry heat | 3 oz | 0.9 |
| Fish, salmon, chinook, smoked | 3 oz | 0.1 |
| Fish, salmon, pink, canned, solids with bone and liquid | 3 oz | 0.3 |
| Fish, sardine, Atlantic, canned in oil, drained solids with bone | 3 oz | 2.2 |
| Fish, tuna, light, canned in oil, drained solids | 3 oz | 37.4 |
| Fish, tuna, light, canned in water, drained solids | 3 oz | 0.2 |
| Fish, tuna, white, canned in water, drained solids | 3 oz | 2.1 |

| | | |
|---|---|---|
| Frankfurter, beef | 1 frank | 0.8 |
| Frankfurter, beef and pork | 1 frank | 0.8 |
| Frankfurter, chicken | 1 frank | 0.0 |
| Frostings, vanilla, creamy, ready-to-eat | 1/12 package | 4.9 |
| Frozen novelties, fruit and juice bars | 1 bar (2.5 fl oz) | 0.7 |
| Frozen novelties, ice type, pop | 1 bar (2 fl oz) | 0.0 |
| Frozen yogurts, vanilla, soft-serve | 1/2 cup | 0.2 |
| Fruit butters, apple | 1 tbsp | 0.0 |
| Fruit cocktail, (peach and pineapple and pear and grape and cherry), canned, heavy syrup, solids and liquids | 1 cup | 6.4 |
| Fruit cocktail, (peach and pineapple and pear and grape and cherry), canned, juice pack, solids and liquids | 1 cup | 6.2 |
| Fruit punch drink, with added nutrients, canned | 8 fl oz | 0.0 |
| Garlic, raw | 1 clove | 0.0 |
| Gelatin desserts, dry mix, prepared with water | 1/2 cup | 0.0 |
| Gelatin desserts, dry mix, reduced calorie, with aspartame, prepared with water | 1/2 cup | 0.0 |
| Grape drink, canned | 8 fl oz | 0.0 |
| Grape juice, canned or bottled, unsweetened, without added vitamin C | 1 cup | 1.0 |
| Grape juice, frozen concentrate, sweetened, | 1 cup | 1.0 |

| | | |
|---|---|---|
| diluted with 3 volume water, with added vitamin C | | |
| Grape juice, frozen concentrate, sweetened, undiluted, with added vitamin C | 6-fl-oz can | 3.0 |
| Grapefruit juice, white, canned, sweetened | 1 cup | 0.0 |
| Grapefruit juice, white, canned, unsweetened | 1 cup | 0.0 |
| Grapefruit juice, white, frozen concentrate, unsweetened, diluted with 3 volume water | 1 cup | 0.0 |
| Grapefruit juice, white, frozen concentrate, unsweetened, undiluted | 6-fl-oz can | 0.2 |
| Grapefruit juice, white, raw | 1 cup | 0.0 |
| Grapefruit, raw, pink and red, all areas | 1/2 grapefruit | 0.0 |
| Grapefruit, raw, white, all areas | 1/2 grapefruit | 0.0 |
| Grapefruit, sections, canned, light syrup pack, solids and liquids | 1 cup | 0.0 |
| Grapes, red or green (european type varieties, such as, Thompson seedless), raw | 1 cup | 23.4 |
| Grapes, red or green (european type varieties, such as, Thompson seedless), raw | 10 grapes | 7.3 |
| Gravy, beef, canned | 1/4 cup | 0.1 |
| Gravy, chicken, canned | 1/4 cup | 0.1 |
| Gravy, turkey, canned | 1/4 cup | 0.0 |
| Ham, chopped, not canned | 2 slices | 0.0 |
| Ham, sliced, extra lean | 2 slices | 0.0 |

| | | |
|---|---|---|
| Ham, sliced, regular (approximately 11% fat) | 2 slices | 0.0 |
| HEALTHY CHOICE Beef Macaroni, frozen entree | 1 package | 4.8 |
| Honey | 1 tbsp | 0.0 |
| Horseradish, prepared | 1 tsp | 0.1 |
| Ice creams, chocolate | 1/2 cup | 0.2 |
| Ice creams, french vanilla, soft-serve | 1/2 cup | 0.8 |
| Ice creams, vanilla | 1/2 cup | 0.2 |
| Ice creams, vanilla, light | 1/2 cup | 0.3 |
| Ice creams, vanilla, rich | 1/2 cup | 1.0 |
| Jams and preserves | 1 tbsp | 0.0 |
| Jellies | 1 tbsp | 0.1 |
| Jerusalem-artichokes, raw | 1 cup | 0.2 |
| Kale, cooked, boiled, drained, without salt | 1 cup | 1062.1 |
| Kale, frozen, cooked, boiled, drained, without salt | 1 cup | 1146.6 |
| Kiwi fruit, (chinese gooseberries), fresh, raw | 1 medium | 30.6 |
| Kohlrabi, cooked, boiled, drained, without salt | 1 cup | 0.2 |
| Lamb, domestic, leg, whole (shank and sirloin), separable lean and fat, trimmed to 1/4" fat, choice, cooked, roasted | 3 oz | 3.6 |
| Lamb, domestic, leg, whole (shank and sirloin), separable lean only, trimmed to 1/4" fat, choice, cooked, roasted | 3 oz | 3.1 |
| Lamb, domestic, loin, separable lean and fat, trimmed to 1/4" fat, choice, cooked, broiled | 3 oz | 4.1 |

| | | |
|---|---|---|
| Lamb, domestic, loin, separable lean only, trimmed to 1/4" fat, choice, cooked, broiled | 3 oz | 3.3 |
| Lard | 1 tbsp | 0.0 |
| Leavening agents, baking powder, double-acting, sodium aluminum sulfate | 1 tsp | 0.0 |
| Leavening agents, baking powder, double-acting, straight phosphate | 1 tsp | 0.0 |
| Leavening agents, baking powder, low-sodium | 1 tsp | 0.0 |
| Leavening agents, baking soda | 1 tsp | 0.0 |
| Leavening agents, cream of tartar | 1 tsp | 0.0 |
| Leavening agents, yeast, baker's, active dry | 1 tsp | 0.0 |
| Leavening agents, yeast, baker's, active dry | 1 pkg | 0.0 |
| Leavening agents, yeast, baker's, compressed | 1 cake | 0.0 |
| Lemon juice, canned or bottled | 1 cup | 0.0 |
| Lemon juice, canned or bottled | 1 tbsp | 0.0 |
| Lemon juice, raw | juice of 1 lemon | 0.0 |
| Lemonade, frozen concentrate, white, prepared with water | 8 fl oz | 0.0 |
| Lemonade, low calorie, with aspartame, powder, prepared with water | 8 fl oz | 0.0 |
| Lemons, raw, without peel | 1 lemon | 0.0 |
| Lentils, mature seeds, cooked, | 1 cup | 3.4 |

| | | |
|---|---|---|
| boiled, without salt | | |
| Lettuce, butterhead (includes boston and bibb types), raw | 1 head | 166.7 |
| Lettuce, butterhead (includes boston and bibb types), raw | 1 medium leaf | 7.7 |
| Lettuce, cos or romaine, raw | 1 leaf | 10.3 |
| Lettuce, cos or romaine, raw | 1 cup | 57.4 |
| Lettuce, green leaf, raw | 1 leaf | 17.4 |
| Lettuce, green leaf, raw | 1 cup | 97.2 |
| Lettuce, iceberg (includes crisphead types), raw | 1 head | 129.9 |
| Lettuce, iceberg (includes crisphead types), raw | 1 medium | 1.9 |
| Lettuce, iceberg (includes crisphead types), raw | 1 cup | 13.3 |
| Lima beans, immature seeds, frozen, baby, cooked, boiled, drained, without salt | 1 cup | 9.4 |
| Lima beans, immature seeds, frozen, fordhook, cooked, boiled, drained, without salt | 1 cup | 8.7 |
| Lima beans, large, mature seeds, cooked, boiled, without salt | 1 cup | 3.8 |
| Lime juice, canned or bottled, unsweetened | 1 tbsp | 0.1 |
| Lime juice, canned or bottled, unsweetened | 1 cup | 1.2 |
| Lime juice, raw | juice of 1 lime | 0.2 |
| Macaroni and Cheese, canned entree | 1 cup | 0.5 |
| Macaroni, cooked, enriched | 1 cup | 0.0 |
| Malted drink mix, chocolate, | 3 | 0.6 |

| | | |
|---|---|---|
| with added nutrients, powder | heaping tsp | |
| Malted drink mix, chocolate, with added nutrients, powder, prepared with whole milk | 1 cup | 0.8 |
| Malted drink mix, natural, with added nutrients, powder | 4-5 heaping tsp | 0.2 |
| Malted drink mix, natural, with added nutrients, powder, prepared with whole milk | 1 cup | 1.1 |
| Mangos, raw | 1 cup | 6.9 |
| Mangos, raw | 1 mango | 8.7 |
| Margarine, regular, tub, composite, 80% fat, with salt | 1 tbsp | 13.2 |
| Margarine, regular, unspecified oils, with salt added | 1 tbsp | 13.1 |
| Margarine, vegetable oil spread, 60% fat, stick | 1 tsp | 4.9 |
| Margarine, vegetable oil spread, 60% fat, stick | 1 tbsp | 14.5 |
| Margarine, vegetable oil spread, 60% fat, tub/bottle | 1 tsp | 4.9 |
| Margarine-butter blend, 60% corn oil margarine and 40% butter | 1 tbsp | 14.7 |
| Margarine-like spread, (approximately 40% fat), unspecified oils | 1 tsp | 4.5 |
| Melons, cantaloupe, raw | 1 cup | 4.0 |
| Melons, cantaloupe, raw | 1/8 melon | 1.7 |
| Melons, honeydew, raw | 1/8 melon | 4.6 |

| | | |
|---|---|---|
| Melons, honeydew, raw | 1 cup | 4.9 |
| Milk shakes, thick chocolate | 10.6 fl oz | 0.6 |
| Milk shakes, thick vanilla | 11 fl oz | 0.6 |
| Milk, buttermilk, dried | 1 tbsp | 0.0 |
| Milk, buttermilk, fluid, cultured, lowfat | 1 cup | 0.2 |
| Milk, canned, condensed, sweetened | 1 cup | 1.8 |
| Milk, canned, evaporated, nonfat | 1 cup | 0.0 |
| Milk, canned, evaporated, without added vitamin A | 1 cup | 1.3 |
| Milk, chocolate, fluid, commercial, lowfat | 1 cup | 0.3 |
| Milk, chocolate, fluid, commercial, reduced fat | 1 cup | 0.5 |
| Milk, chocolate, fluid, commercial, whole | 1 cup | 0.5 |
| Milk, dry, nonfat, instant, with added vitamin A | 1/3 cup | 0.0 |
| Milk, lowfat, fluid, 1% milkfat, with added vitamin A | 1 cup | 0.2 |
| Milk, nonfat, fluid, with added vitamin A (fat free or skim) | 1 cup | 0.0 |
| Milk, reduced fat, fluid, 2% milkfat, with added vitamin A | 1 cup | 0.5 |
| Milk, whole, 3.25% milkfat | 1 cup | 0.5 |
| Miso | 1 cup | 20.7 |
| Mollusks, clam, mixed species, canned, drained solids | 3 oz | 0.3 |
| Mollusks, clam, mixed species, raw | 3 oz | 0.2 |
| Mollusks, oyster, eastern, wild, raw | 6 medium | 0.1 |
| Muffins, blueberry, | 1 muffin | 3.1 |

| commercially prepared | | |
|---|---|---|
| Muffins, corn, commercially prepared | 1 muffin | 1.3 |
| Muffins, oat bran | 1 muffin | 7.4 |
| Muffins, wheat bran, toaster-type with raisins, toasted | 1 muffin | 5.9 |
| Mung beans, mature seeds, sprouted, cooked, boiled, drained, without salt | 1 cup | 28.1 |
| Mung beans, mature seeds, sprouted, raw | 1 cup | 34.3 |
| Mushrooms, canned, drained solids | 1 cup | 0.2 |
| Mushrooms, cooked, boiled, drained, without salt | 1 cup | 0.2 |
| Mushrooms, raw | 1 cup | 0.0 |
| Mushrooms, shiitake, cooked, without salt | 1 cup | 0.1 |
| Mushrooms, shiitake, dried | 1 mushroom | 0.0 |
| Mustard greens, cooked, boiled, drained, without salt | 1 cup | 419.3 |
| Mustard, prepared, yellow | 1 tsp or 1 packet | 0.1 |
| Nectarines, raw | 1 nectarine | 3.0 |
| Noodles, chinese, chow mein | 1 cup | 3.0 |
| Noodles, egg, cooked, enriched | 1 cup | 0.0 |
| Noodles, egg, spinach, cooked, enriched | 1 cup | 161.8 |
| Nuts, almonds | 1 oz (24 nuts) | 0.0 |
| Nuts, brazilnuts, dried, | 1 oz (6-8 | 0.0 |

| unblanched | nuts) | |
|---|---|---|
| Nuts, cashew nuts, dry roasted, with salt added | 1 oz | 9.8 |
| Nuts, cashew nuts, oil roasted, with salt added | 1 oz (18 nuts) | 9.8 |
| Nuts, chestnuts, european, roasted | 1 cup | 11.2 |
| Nuts, coconut meat, dried (desiccated), sweetened, shredded | 1 cup | 0.3 |
| Nuts, coconut meat, raw | 1 piece | 0.1 |
| Nuts, hazelnuts or filberts | 1 oz | 4.0 |
| Nuts, macadamia nuts, dry roasted, with salt added | 1 oz (10-12 nuts) | 0.0 |
| Nuts, mixed nuts, dry roasted, with peanuts, with salt added | 1 oz | 3.7 |
| Nuts, mixed nuts, oil roasted, with peanuts, with salt added | 1 oz | 3.6 |
| Nuts, pecans | 1 oz (20 halves) | 1.0 |
| Nuts, pine nuts, dried | 1 oz | 15.3 |
| Nuts, pine nuts, dried | 1 tbsp | 4.6 |
| Nuts, pistachio nuts, dry roasted, with salt added | 1 oz (47 nuts) | 3.7 |
| Nuts, walnuts, english | 1 oz (14 halves) | 0.8 |
| Oat bran, raw | 1 cup | 3.0 |
| Oil, olive, salad or cooking | 1 tbsp | 8.1 |
| Oil, peanut, salad or cooking | 1 tbsp | 0.1 |
| Oil, sesame, salad or cooking | 1 tbsp | 1.8 |
| Oil, soybean, salad or cooking, (hydrogenated) | 1 tbsp | 3.4 |
| Oil, soybean, salad or cooking, (hydrogenated) and cottonseed | 1 tbsp | 3.4 |

| | | |
|---|---|---|
| Oil, vegetable safflower, salad or cooking, oleic, over 70% (primary safflower oil of commerce) | 1 tbsp | 1.0 |
| Oil, vegetable, corn, industrial and retail, all purpose salad or cooking | 1 tbsp | 0.3 |
| Oil, vegetable, sunflower, linoleic, (approx. 65%) | 1 tbsp | 0.7 |
| Okra, cooked, boiled, drained, without salt | 1 cup | 64.0 |
| Okra, frozen, cooked, boiled, drained, without salt | 1 cup | 88.0 |
| Olives, ripe, canned (small-extra large) | 5 large | 0.3 |
| Onions, cooked, boiled, drained, without salt | 1 medium | 0.5 |
| Onions, cooked, boiled, drained, without salt | 1 cup | 1.1 |
| Onions, dehydrated flakes | 1 tbsp | 0.2 |
| Onions, raw | 1 slice | 0.1 |
| Onions, raw | 1 whole | 0.4 |
| Onions, raw | 1 cup | 0.6 |
| Onions, spring or scallions (includes tops and bulb), raw | 1 whole | 31.1 |
| Onions, spring or scallions (includes tops and bulb), raw | 1 cup | 207.0 |
| Orange juice, canned, unsweetened | 1 cup | 0.2 |
| Orange juice, frozen concentrate, unsweetened, diluted with 3 volume water | 1 cup | 0.2 |
| Orange juice, frozen concentrate, unsweetened, undiluted | 6-fl-oz can | 0.9 |

| | | |
|---|---|---|
| Orange juice, raw | juice from 1 orange | 0.1 |
| Orange juice, raw | 1 cup | 0.2 |
| Oranges, raw, all commercial varieties | 1 cup | 0.0 |
| Oranges, raw, all commercial varieties | 1 orange | 0.0 |
| Pancakes plain, frozen, ready-to-heat (includes buttermilk) | 1 pancake | 2.3 |
| Papayas, raw | 1 cup | 3.6 |
| Papayas, raw | 1 papaya | 7.9 |
| Parsley, raw | 10 sprigs | 164.0 |
| Parsnips, cooked, boiled, drained, without salt | 1 cup | 1.6 |
| Pasta with meatballs in tomato sauce, canned entree | 1 cup | 4.5 |
| Peaches, canned, heavy syrup pack, solids and liquids | 1 cup | 4.5 |
| Peaches, canned, heavy syrup pack, solids and liquids | 1 half | 1.7 |
| Peaches, canned, juice pack, solids and liquids | 1 cup | 4.2 |
| Peaches, canned, juice pack, solids and liquids | 1 half | 1.7 |
| Peaches, dried, sulfured, uncooked | 3 halves | 6.1 |
| Peaches, frozen, sliced, sweetened | 1 cup | 5.5 |
| Peaches, raw | 1 cup | 4.4 |
| Peaches, raw | 1 peach | 2.5 |
| Peanut butter, chunk style, with salt | 1 tbsp | 0.1 |
| Peanut butter, smooth style, with salt | 1 tbsp | 0.1 |
| Peanuts, all types, dry- | 1 oz | 0.0 |

| | | |
|---|---|---|
| roasted, with salt | (approx 28) | |
| Peanuts, all types, dry-roasted, without salt | 1 oz (approx 28) | 0.0 |
| Peanuts, all types, oil-roasted, with salt | 1 oz | 0.0 |
| Pears, asian, raw | 1 pear | 12.4 |
| Pears, asian, raw | 1 pear | 5.5 |
| Pears, canned, heavy syrup pack, solids and liquids | 1 cup | 0.8 |
| Pears, canned, heavy syrup pack, solids and liquids | 1 half | 0.2 |
| Pears, canned, juice pack, solids and liquids | 1 half | 0.2 |
| Pears, canned, juice pack, solids and liquids | 1 cup | 0.7 |
| Pears, raw | 1 pear | 7.5 |
| Peas, edible-podded, boiled, drained, without salt | 1 cup | 40.0 |
| Peas, edible-podded, frozen, cooked, boiled, drained, without salt | 1 cup | 48.3 |
| Peas, green, canned, regular pack, drained solids | 1 cup | 36.4 |
| Peas, green, frozen, cooked, boiled, drained, without salt | 1 cup | 38.4 |
| Peas, split, mature seeds, cooked, boiled, without salt | 1 cup | 9.8 |
| Peppers, hot chili, green, raw | 1 pepper | 6.4 |
| Peppers, hot chili, red, raw | 1 pepper | 6.3 |
| Peppers, jalapeno, canned, solids and liquids | 1/4 cup | 3.4 |
| Peppers, sweet, green, cooked, boiled, drained, | 1 cup | 12.9 |

| without salt | | |
|---|---|---|
| Peppers, sweet, green, raw | 1 cup | 11.0 |
| Peppers, sweet, green, raw | 1 ring | 0.7 |
| Peppers, sweet, green, raw | 1 pepper | 8.8 |
| Peppers, sweet, red, cooked, boiled, drained, without salt | 1 cup | 6.9 |
| Peppers, sweet, red, raw | 1 pepper | 5.8 |
| Peppers, sweet, red, raw | 1 cup | 7.3 |
| Pickle relish, sweet | 1 tbsp | 12.5 |
| Pickles, cucumber, dill | 1 pickle | 11.9 |
| Pie crust, cookie-type, prepared from recipe, graham cracker, baked | 1 pie shell | 59.0 |
| Pie crust, standard-type, frozen, ready-to-bake, baked | 1 pie shell | 10.3 |
| Pie crust, standard-type, prepared from recipe, baked | 1 pie shell | 26.6 |
| Pie fillings, apple, canned | 1/8 of 21-oz can | 0.0 |
| Pie, apple, commercially prepared, enriched flour | 1 piece | 4.1 |
| Pie, blueberry, commercially prepared | 1 piece | 12.3 |
| Pie, cherry, commercially prepared | 1 piece | 8.9 |
| Pie, fried pies, fruit | 1 pie | 5.2 |
| Pie, lemon meringue, commercially prepared | 1 piece | 2.4 |
| Pie, pecan, commercially prepared | 1 piece | 5.4 |
| Pie, pumpkin, commercially prepared | 1 piece | 6.8 |
| Pimento, canned | 1 tbsp | 1.0 |
| Pineapple and grapefruit juice drink, canned | 8 fl oz | 0.3 |

| | | |
|---|---|---|
| Pineapple and orange juice drink, canned | 8 fl oz | 0.3 |
| Pineapple juice, canned, unsweetened, without added ascorbic acid | 1 cup | 0.8 |
| Pineapple, canned, heavy syrup pack, solids and liquids | 1 cup | 0.8 |
| Pineapple, canned, heavy syrup pack, solids and liquids | 1 slice | 0.1 |
| Pineapple, canned, juice pack, solids and liquids | 1 slice | 0.1 |
| Pineapple, canned, juice pack, solids and liquids | 1 cup | 0.7 |
| Pineapple, raw, all varieties | 1 cup | 1.1 |
| Pizza, cheese topping, regular crust, frozen, cooked | 1 serving | 4.2 |
| Plantains, cooked | 1 cup | 1.1 |
| Plantains, raw | 1 medium | 1.3 |
| Plums, canned, purple, heavy syrup pack, solids and liquids | 1 plum | 2.0 |
| Plums, canned, purple, heavy syrup pack, solids and liquids | 1 cup | 11.1 |
| Plums, canned, purple, juice pack, solids and liquids | 1 plum | 2.0 |
| Plums, canned, purple, juice pack, solids and liquids | 1 cup | 10.8 |
| Plums, dried (prunes), stewed, without added sugar | 1 cup | 64.7 |
| Plums, dried (prunes), uncooked | 5 prunes | 25.0 |
| Plums, raw | 1 plum | 4.2 |
| Pork and beef sausage, fresh, cooked | 2 links | 0.4 |
| Pork Sausage, Fresh, Cooked | 1 patty | 0.1 |

| | | |
|---|---|---|
| Pork Sausage, Fresh, Cooked | 2 links | 0.1 |
| Pork, cured, bacon, cooked, broiled, pan-fried or roasted | 3 medium slices | 0.0 |
| Pork, cured, canadian-style bacon, grilled | 2 slices | 0.0 |
| Pork, cured, ham, extra lean and regular, canned, roasted | 3 oz | 0.0 |
| Pork, cured, ham, whole, separable lean and fat, roasted | 3 oz | 0.0 |
| Pork, cured, ham, whole, separable lean only, roasted | 3 oz | 0.0 |
| Pork, fresh, leg (ham), whole, separable lean and fat, cooked, roasted | 3 oz | 0.0 |
| Pork, fresh, leg (ham), whole, separable lean only, cooked, roasted | 3 oz | 0.0 |
| Pork, fresh, loin, center loin (chops), bone-in, separable lean and fat, cooked, pan-fried | 3 oz | 0.0 |
| Pork, fresh, loin, center loin (chops), bone-in, separable lean only, cooked, pan-fried | 3 oz | 0.0 |
| Pork, fresh, shoulder, arm picnic, separable lean and fat, cooked, braised | 3 oz | 0.0 |
| Pork, fresh, shoulder, arm picnic, separable lean only, cooked, braised | 3 oz | 0.0 |
| Pork, fresh, spareribs, separable lean and fat, cooked, braised | 3 oz | 0.0 |
| Potato pancakes | 1 pancake | 2.1 |

| | | |
|---|---|---|
| Potato puffs, frozen, oven-heated | 10 puffs | 3.2 |
| Potato, baked, flesh and skin, without salt | 1 potato | 4.0 |
| Potatoes, baked, flesh, without salt | 1 potato | 0.5 |
| Potatoes, baked, skin, without salt | 1 skin | 1.0 |
| Potatoes, boiled, cooked in skin, flesh, without salt | 1 potato | 2.9 |
| Potatoes, boiled, cooked without skin, flesh, without salt | 1 cup | 3.3 |
| Potatoes, boiled, cooked without skin, flesh, without salt | 1 potato | 2.8 |
| Potatoes, french fried, all types, salt added in processing, frozen, home prepared, oven heated | 10 strips | 1.3 |
| Potatoes, hashed brown, frozen, plain, prepared | 1 patty | 1.1 |
| Potatoes, hashed brown, home-prepared | 1 cup | 5.8 |
| Potatoes, mashed, dehydrated, prepared from flakes without milk, whole milk and butter added | 1 cup | 3.2 |
| Potatoes, mashed, home-prepared, whole milk added | 1 cup | 3.8 |
| Potatoes, mashed, home-prepared, whole milk and margarine added | 1 cup | 12.6 |
| Poultry food products, ground turkey, cooked | 1 patty | 0.7 |
| Prune juice, canned | 1 cup | 8.7 |
| Puddings, chocolate, ready-to- | 4 oz | 1.1 |

| eat | | |
|---|---|---|
| Puddings, tapioca, ready-to-eat | 4 oz | 1.0 |
| Puddings, vanilla, ready-to-eat | 4 oz | 0.0 |
| Pumpkin, canned, without salt | 1 cup | 39.2 |
| Pumpkin, cooked, boiled, drained, without salt | 1 cup | 2.0 |
| Radishes, raw | 1 radish | 0.1 |
| Raisins, seedless | 1 cup | 5.1 |
| Raisins, seedless | 1 packet | 0.5 |
| Raspberries, frozen, red, sweetened | 1 cup | 16.3 |
| Raspberries, raw | 1 cup | 9.6 |
| Refried beans, canned (includes USDA commodity) | 1 cup | 6.0 |
| Rhubarb, frozen, cooked, with sugar | 1 cup | 71.0 |
| Rice, brown, long-grain, cooked | 1 cup | 1.2 |
| Rice, white, long-grain, parboiled, enriched, cooked | 1 cup | 0.0 |
| Rice, white, long-grain, parboiled, enriched, dry | 1 cup | 0.2 |
| Rice, white, long-grain, precooked or instant, enriched, prepared | 1 cup | 0.0 |
| Rice, white, long-grain, regular, cooked | 1 cup | 0.0 |
| Rice, white, long-grain, regular, raw, enriched | 1 cup | 0.2 |
| Rolls, dinner, plain, commercially prepared (includes brown-and-serve) | 1 roll | 0.8 |
| Rolls, hamburger or hotdog, plain | 1 roll | 1.3 |

| | | |
|---|---|---|
| Rolls, hard (includes kaiser) | 1 roll | 0.3 |
| Rutabagas, cooked, boiled, drained, without salt | 1 cup | 0.5 |
| Salad dressing, blue or roquefort cheese dressing, commercial, regular | 1 tbsp | 13.9 |
| Salad dressing, french dressing, commercial, regular | 1 tbsp | 18.9 |
| Salad dressing, french dressing, reduced fat | 1 tbsp | 0.8 |
| Salad dressing, home recipe, cooked | 1 tbsp | 2.2 |
| Salad dressing, home recipe, vinegar and oil | 1 tbsp | 15.4 |
| Salad dressing, italian dressing, commercial, regular | 1 tbsp | 8.2 |
| Salad dressing, italian dressing, reduced fat | 1 tbsp | 1.9 |
| Salad dressing, mayonnaise, soybean oil, with salt | 1 tbsp | 5.8 |
| Salad dressing, russian dressing | 1 tbsp | 8.2 |
| Salad dressing, russian dressing, low calorie | 1 tbsp | 1.1 |
| Salad dressing, thousand island dressing, reduced fat | 1 tbsp | 4.2 |
| Salad dressing, thousand island, commercial, regular | 1 tbsp | 10.8 |
| Salami, cooked, beef and pork | 2 slices | 0.7 |
| Salami, dry or hard, pork, beef | 2 slices | 0.3 |
| Salt, table | 1 tsp | 0.0 |
| Sandwich spread, pork, beef | 1 tbsp | 0.2 |
| Sauce, barbecue sauce | 1 tbsp | 0.0 |
| Sauce, hoisin, ready-to-serve | 1 tbsp | 0.1 |
| Sauce, homemade, white, | 1 cup | 2.3 |

| | | |
|---|---|---|
| medium | | |
| Sauce, pasta, spaghetti/marinara, ready-to-serve | 1 cup | 34.8 |
| Sauce, ready-to-serve, pepper or hot | 1 tsp | 0.1 |
| Sauce, ready-to-serve, salsa | 1 tbsp | 0.7 |
| Sauce, teriyaki, ready-to-serve | 1 tbsp | 0.0 |
| Sauerkraut, canned, solids and liquids | 1 cup | 135.0 |
| Sausage, Vienna, canned, chicken, beef, pork | 1 sausage | 0.3 |
| Seaweed, kelp, raw | 2 tbsp | 6.6 |
| Seaweed, spirulina, dried | 1 tbsp | 0.2 |
| Seeds, pumpkin and squash seed kernels, roasted, with salt added | 1 oz (142 seeds) | 13.4 |
| Seeds, sesame butter, tahini, from roasted and toasted kernels (most common type) | 1 tbsp | 0.0 |
| Seeds, sesame seed kernels, dried (decorticated) | 1 tbsp | 0.0 |
| Seeds, sunflower seed kernels, dry roasted, with salt added | 1/4 cup | 0.9 |
| Seeds, sunflower seed kernels, dry roasted, with salt added | 1 oz | 0.8 |
| Shake, fast food, chocolate | 16 fl oz | 5.0 |
| Shake, fast food, vanilla | 16 fl oz | 1.3 |
| Sherbet, orange | 1/2 cup | 0.0 |
| Shortening, household, soybean (hydrogenated)-cottonseed (hydrogenated) | 1 tbsp | 5.5 |
| Snacks, beef jerky, chopped | 1 large | 0.5 |

| | | |
|---|---|---|
| and formed | piece | |
| Snacks, corn-based, extruded, chips, plain | 1 oz | 1.8 |
| Snacks, corn-based, extruded, puffs or twists, cheese-flavor | 1 oz | 10.2 |
| Snacks, fruit leather, pieces | 1 oz | 5.2 |
| Snacks, fruit leather, rolls | 1 large | 3.8 |
| Snacks, oriental mix, rice-based | 1 oz (about 1/4 cup) | 0.7 |
| Snacks, popcorn, air-popped | 1 cup | 0.1 |
| Snacks, popcorn, cakes | 1 cake | 0.1 |
| Snacks, popcorn, caramel-coated, with peanuts | 1 cup | 1.6 |
| Snacks, popcorn, caramel-coated, without peanuts | 1 cup | 4.4 |
| Snacks, popcorn, oil-popped, microwaved | 1 cup | 1.7 |
| Snacks, pork skins, plain | 1 oz | 0.0 |
| Snacks, potato chips, made from dried potatoes, light | 1 oz | 2.0 |
| Snacks, potato chips, made from dried potatoes, plain | 1 oz | 2.0 |
| Snacks, potato chips, plain, salted | 1 oz | 6.3 |
| Snacks, potato chips, plain, unsalted | 1 oz | 6.3 |
| Snacks, potato chips, reduced fat | 1 oz | 3.8 |
| Snacks, pretzels, hard, plain, salted | 10 pretzels | 0.5 |
| Snacks, rice cakes, brown rice, plain | 1 cake | 0.2 |
| Snacks, tortilla chips, plain, white corn | 1 oz | 0.2 |

| | | |
|---|---|---|
| Snacks,tortilla chips, nacho-flavor | 1 oz | 0.4 |
| Soup, bean with pork, canned, prepared with equal volume water, commercial | 1 cup | 3.0 |
| Soup, beef broth or bouillon, powder, dry | 1 packet | 0.2 |
| Soup, beef noodle, canned, prepared with equal volume water, commercial | 1 cup | 1.2 |
| Soup, chicken noodle, canned, chunky, ready-toserve | 1 cup | 3.8 |
| Soup, chicken noodle, canned, prepared with equal volume water, commercial | 1 cup | 0.0 |
| Soup, chicken noodle, dehydrated, prepared with water | 1 cup | 3.5 |
| Soup, chicken with rice, canned, prepared with equal volume water, commercial | 1 cup | 0.5 |
| Soup, clam chowder, manhattan, canned, prepared with equal volume water | 1 cup | 7.1 |
| Soup, clam chowder, new england, canned, prepared with equal volume milk, commercial | 1 cup | 2.2 |
| Soup, cream of mushroom, canned, prepared with equal volume milk, commercial | 1 cup | 2.7 |
| Soup, cream of mushroom, canned, prepared with equal volume water, commercial | 1 cup | 2.0 |
| Soup, onion mix, dehydrated, dry form | 1 packet | 0.5 |

| | | |
|---|---|---|
| Soup, onion, dehydrated, prepared with water | 1 cup | 0.2 |
| Soup, pea, green, canned, prepared with equal volume water, commercial | 1 cup | 7.3 |
| Soup, stock, fish, home-prepared | 1 cup | 0.0 |
| Soup, tomato, canned, prepared with equal volume milk, commercial | 1 cup | 2.5 |
| Soup, tomato, canned, prepared with equal volume water, commercial | 1 cup | 3.9 |
| Soup, vegetable beef, prepared with equal volume water, commercial | 1 cup | 4.4 |
| Soup, vegetable, canned, chunky, ready-to-serve, commercial | 1 cup | 19.4 |
| Soup, vegetarian vegetable, canned, prepared with equal volume water, commercial | 1 cup | 6.3 |
| Sour dressing, non-butterfat, cultured, filled cream-type | 1 tbsp | 0.5 |
| Soy milk, fluid | 1 cup | 7.4 |
| Soy sauce made from soy and wheat (shoyu) | 1 tbsp | 0.0 |
| Soybeans, mature cooked, boiled, without salt | 1 cup | 33.0 |
| Spaghetti with meat sauce, frozen entree | 1 package | 2.0 |
| Spaghetti, cooked, enriched, without added salt | 1 cup | 0.0 |
| Spaghetti, whole-wheat, cooked | 1 cup | 1.0 |

| | | |
|---|---|---|
| Spices, celery seed | 1 tsp | 0.0 |
| Spices, chili powder | 1 tsp | 2.7 |
| Spices, cinnamon, ground | 1 tsp | 0.7 |
| Spices, curry powder | 1 tsp | 2.0 |
| Spices, garlic powder | 1 tsp | 0.0 |
| Spices, onion powder | 1 tsp | 0.1 |
| Spices, oregano, dried | 1 tsp | 9.3 |
| Spices, paprika | 1 tsp | 1.7 |
| Spices, parsley, dried | 1 tbsp | 17.7 |
| Spices, pepper, black | 1 tsp | 3.4 |
| Spinach souffle | 136 | 1 cup |
| Spinach, canned, drained solids | 214 | 1 cup |
| Spinach, cooked, boiled, drained, without salt | 1 cup | 888.5 |
| Spinach, frozen, chopped or leaf, cooked, boiled, drained, without salt | 1 cup | 1027.3 |
| Spinach, raw | 1 cup | 144.9 |
| Spinach, raw | 1 leaf | 48.3 |
| Squash, summer, all varieties, cooked, boiled, drained, without salt | 1 cup | 6.3 |
| Squash, summer, all varieties, raw | 1 cup | 3.4 |
| Squash, winter, all varieties, cooked, baked, without salt | 1 cup | 9.0 |
| Strawberries, frozen, sweetened, sliced | 1 cup | 4.3 |
| Strawberries, raw | 1 cup | 3.7 |
| Strawberries, raw | 1 strawberry | 0.4 |
| Strawberries, raw | 1 strawberr | 0.3 |

|  | y |  |
|---|---|---|
| Sugars, brown | 1 tsp | 0.0 |
| Sugars, granulated | 1 tsp | 0.0 |
| Sugars, powdered | 1 tbsp | 0.0 |
| Sweet potato, canned, syrup pack, drained solids | 1 cup | 5.1 |
| Sweet potato, canned, vacuum pack | 1 cup | 5.6 |
| Sweet potato, cooked, baked in skin, without salt | 1 potato | 3.4 |
| Sweet potato, cooked, boiled, without skin | 1 potato | 3.3 |
| Sweet rolls, cinnamon, commercially prepared with raisins | 1 roll | 2.6 |
| Syrups, chocolate, fudge-type | 1 tbsp | 0.4 |
| Syrups, corn, light | 1 tbsp | 0.0 |
| Syrups, maple | 1 tbsp | 0.0 |
| Syrups, table blends, pancake | 1 tbsp | 0.0 |
| Syrups, table blends, pancake, reduced-calorie | 1 tbsp | 0.0 |
| Taco shells, baked | 1 medium | 0.7 |
| Tangerine juice, canned, sweetened | 1 cup | 0.0 |
| Tangerines, (mandarin oranges), canned, light syrup pack | 1 cup | 0.0 |
| Tangerines, (mandarin oranges), raw | 1 tangerine | 0.0 |
| Tapioca, pearl, dry | 1 cup | 0.0 |
| Tea, brewed, prepared with tap water | 6 fl oz | 0.0 |
| Tea, herb, chamomile, brewed | 6 fl oz | 0.0 |
| Tea, herb, other than | 6 fl oz | 0.0 |

| | | |
|---|---|---|
| chamomile, brewed | | |
| Tea, instant, sweetened with sodium saccharin, lemon-flavored, prepared | 8 fl oz | 0.0 |
| Tea, instant, sweetened with sugar, lemon-flavored, without added ascorbic acid, powder, prepared | 8 fl oz | 0.0 |
| Tea, instant, unsweetened, powder, prepared | 8 fl oz | 0.0 |
| Toaster pastries, fruit (includes apple, blueberry, cherry, strawberry) | 1 pastry | 2.1 |
| Tofu, soft, prepared with calcium sulfate and magnesium chloride (nigari) | 1 piece | 2.4 |
| Tomatillos, raw | 1 medium | 3.3 |
| Tomato juice, canned, with salt added | 1 cup | 5.6 |
| Tomato products, canned, paste, without salt added | 1 cup | 29.9 |
| Tomato products, canned, puree, without salt added | 1 cup | 8.5 |
| Tomato products, canned, sauce | 1 cup | 6.9 |
| Tomatoes, red, ripe, canned, stewed | 1 cup | 6.1 |
| Tomatoes, red, ripe, canned, whole, regular pack | 1 cup | 6.7 |
| Tomatoes, red, ripe, raw, year round average | 1 slice | 1.6 |
| Tomatoes, red, ripe, raw, year round average | 1 cup | 14.2 |
| Tomatoes, red, ripe, raw, year | 1 tomato | 9.7 |

| | | |
|---|---|---|
| round average | | |
| Tomatoes, red, ripe, raw, year round average | 1 cherry tomato | 1.3 |
| Tomatoes, sun-dried | 1 piece | 0.9 |
| Tortillas, ready-to-bake or -fry, corn | 1 tortilla | 0.0 |
| Tortillas, ready-to-bake or -fry, flour | 1 tortilla | 1.1 |
| Turkey patties, breaded, battered, fried | 1 patty | 13.4 |
| Turkey roast, boneless, frozen, seasoned, light and dark meat, roasted | 3 oz | 0.6 |
| Turkey, all classes, dark meat, cooked, roasted | 3 oz | 3.3 |
| Turkey, all classes, giblets, cooked, simmered, some giblet fat | 1 cup | 0.9 |
| Turkey, all classes, light meat, cooked, roasted | 3 oz | 0.0 |
| Turkey, all classes, meat only, cooked, roasted | 1 cup | 5.2 |
| Turkey, all classes, neck, meat only, cooked, simmered | 1 neck | 5.6 |
| Turnip greens, cooked, boiled, drained, without salt | 1 cup | 529.3 |
| Turnip greens, frozen, cooked, boiled, drained, without salt | 1 cup | 851.0 |
| Turnips, cooked, boiled, drained, without salt | 1 cup | 0.2 |
| Vanilla extract | 1 tsp | 0.0 |
| Veal, leg (top round), separable lean and fat, cooked, braised | 3 oz | 6.0 |
| Vegetable juice cocktail, | 1 cup | 12.8 |

| | | |
|---|---|---|
| canned | | |
| Vegetable oil, canola | 1 tbsp | 17.1 |
| Vegetables, mixed, canned, drained solids | 1 cup | 20.2 |
| Vegetables, mixed, frozen, cooked, boiled, drained, without salt | 1 cup | 29.1 |
| Vinegar, cider | 1 tbsp | 0.0 |
| Waffles, plain, frozen, ready - to-heat, toasted | 1 waffle | 2.2 |
| Water, municipal | 8 fl oz | 0.0 |
| Waterchestnuts, chinese, canned, solids and liquids | 1 cup | 0.3 |
| Watermelon, raw | 1 wedge | 0.3 |
| Watermelon, raw | 1 cup | 0.2 |
| Wheat flour, white, all-purpose, enriched, bleached | 1 cup | 0.4 |
| Wheat flour, white, all-purpose, self-rising, enriched | 1 cup | 0.4 |
| Wheat flour, white, bread, enriched | 1 cup | 0.4 |
| Wheat flour, white, cake, enriched | 1 cup | 0.4 |
| Wheat flour, whole-grain | 1 cup | 2.3 |
| Wild rice, cooked | 1 cup | 0.8 |
| Yogurt, fruit, low fat, 10 grams protein per 8 ounce | 8-oz container | 0.2 |
| Yogurt, plain, low fat, 12 grams protein per 8 ounce | 8-oz container | 0.5 |
| Yogurt, plain, skim milk, 13 grams protein per 8 ounce | 8-oz container | 0.5 |
| Yogurt, plain, whole milk, 8 grams protein per 8 ounce | 8-oz container | 0.5 |

# AMOUNTS OF VITAMIN K
# IN COMMON FOODS
# BY AMOUNT, DESCENDING

| Description | Common Measure | Mcg Vit. K |
|---|---|---|
| Kale, frozen, cooked, boiled, drained, without salt | 1 cup | 1146.6 |
| Kale, cooked, boiled, drained, without salt | 1 cup | 1062.1 |
| Collards, frozen, chopped, cooked, boiled, drained, without salt | 1 cup | 1059.4 |
| Spinach, frozen, chopped or leaf, cooked, boiled, drained, without salt | 1 cup | 1027.3 |
| Spinach, cooked, boiled, drained, without salt | 1 cup | 888.5 |
| Turnip greens, frozen, cooked, boiled, drained, without salt | 1 cup | 851.0 |
| Collards, cooked, boiled, drained, without salt | 1 cup | 836.0 |
| Beet greens, cooked, boiled, drained, without salt | 1 cup | 697.0 |
| Turnip greens, cooked, boiled, drained, without salt | 1 cup | 529.3 |

| | | |
|---|---|---|
| Mustard greens, cooked, boiled, drained, without salt | 1 cup | 419.3 |
| Brussels sprouts, frozen, cooked, boiled, drained, without salt | 1 cup | 299.9 |
| Broccoli, cooked, boiled, drained, without salt | 1 cup | 220.1 |
| Brussels sprouts, cooked, boiled, drained, without salt | 1 cup | 218.9 |
| Onions, spring or scallions (includes tops and bulb), raw | 1 cup | 207.0 |
| Dandelion greens, cooked, boiled, drained, without salt | 1 cup | 203.6 |
| Broccoli, frozen, chopped, cooked, boiled, drained, without salt | 1 cup | 183.1 |
| Lettuce, butterhead (includes boston and bibb types), raw | 1 head | 166.7 |
| Parsley, raw | 10 sprigs | 164.0 |
| Noodles, egg, spinach, cooked, enriched | 1 cup | 161.8 |
| Spinach, raw | 1 cup | 144.9 |
| Asparagus, frozen, cooked, boiled, drained, without salt | 1 cup | 144.0 |
| Sauerkraut, canned, solids and liquids | 1 cup | 135.0 |
| Lettuce, iceberg (includes crisphead types), raw | 1 head | 129.9 |
| Endive, raw | 1 cup | 115.5 |
| Lettuce, green leaf, raw | 1 cup | 97.2 |
| Broccoli, raw | 1 cup | 89.4 |
| Okra, frozen, cooked, boiled, drained, without salt | 1 cup | 88.0 |
| Cabbage, cooked, boiled, drained, without salt | 1 cup | 73.4 |

| | | |
|---|---|---|
| Rhubarb, frozen, cooked, with sugar | 1 cup | 71.0 |
| Plums, dried (prunes), stewed, without added sugar | 1 cup | 64.7 |
| Okra, cooked, boiled, drained, without salt | 1 cup | 64.0 |
| Cowpeas (blackeyes), immature seeds, frozen, cooked, boiled, drained, without salt | 1 cup | 62.6 |
| Pie crust, cookie-type, prepared from recipe, graham cracker, baked | 1 pie shell | 59.0 |
| Cabbage, chinese (pak-choi), cooked, boiled, drained, without salt | 1 cup | 57.8 |
| Lettuce, cos or romaine, raw | 1 cup | 57.4 |
| Celery, cooked, boiled, drained, without salt | 1 cup | 56.7 |
| Fast foods, coleslaw | 3/4 cup | 56.4 |
| Bread crumbs, dry, grated, seasoned | 1 cup | 55.2 |
| Broccoli, cooked, boiled, drained, without salt | 1 spear | 52.2 |
| Cucumber, with peel, raw | 1 large | 49.4 |
| Peas, edible-podded, frozen, cooked, boiled, drained, without salt | 1 cup | 48.3 |
| Spinach, raw | 1 leaf | 48.3 |
| Cabbage, savoy, raw | 1 cup | 48.2 |
| Asparagus, frozen, cooked, boiled, drained, without salt | 4 spears | 48.0 |
| Cowpeas (Blackeyes), immature seeds, cooked, boiled, drained, without salt | 1 cup | 43.9 |

| | | |
|---|---|---|
| Cabbage, raw | 1 cup | 42.0 |
| Blueberries, frozen, sweetened | 1 cup | 40.7 |
| Peas, edible-podded, boiled, drained, without salt | 1 cup | 40.0 |
| Pumpkin, canned, without salt | 1 cup | 39.2 |
| Peas, green, frozen, cooked, boiled, drained, without salt | 1 cup | 38.4 |
| Fish, tuna, light, canned in oil, drained solids | 3 oz | 37.4 |
| Carrot juice, canned | 1 cup | 36.6 |
| Peas, green, canned, regular pack, drained solids | 1 cup | 36.4 |
| Celery, raw | 1 cup | 35.2 |
| Sauce, pasta, spaghetti/marinara, ready-to-serve | 1 cup | 34.8 |
| Mung beans, mature seeds, sprouted, raw | 1 cup | 34.3 |
| Soybeans, mature cooked, boiled, without salt | 1 cup | 33.0 |
| Broccoli, raw | 1 spear | 31.5 |
| Onions, spring or scallions (includes tops and bulb), raw | 1 whole | 31.1 |
| Kiwi fruit, (chinese gooseberries), fresh, raw | 1 medium | 30.6 |
| Asparagus, cooked, boiled, drained | 4 spears | 30.4 |
| Tomato products, canned, paste, without salt added | 1 cup | 29.9 |
| Asparagus, canned, drained solids | 4 spears | 29.7 |
| Vegetables, mixed, frozen, cooked, boiled, drained, | 1 cup | 29.1 |

| | | |
|---|---|---|
| without salt | | |
| Blackberries, raw | 1 cup | 28.5 |
| Mung beans, mature seeds, sprouted, cooked, boiled, drained, without salt | 1 cup | 28.1 |
| Blueberries, raw | 1 cup | 28.0 |
| Cabbage, red, raw | 1 cup | 26.7 |
| Pie crust, standard-type, prepared from recipe, baked | 1 pie shell | 26.6 |
| Plums, dried (prunes), uncooked | 5 prunes | 25.0 |
| Artichokes, (globe or french), cooked, boiled, drained, without salt | 1 cup | 24.9 |
| Grapes, red or green (european type varieties, such as, Thompson seedless), raw | 1 cup | 23.4 |
| Carrots, cooked, boiled, drained, without salt | 1 cup | 21.4 |
| Cauliflower, frozen, cooked, boiled, drained, without salt | 1 cup | 21.4 |
| Miso | 1 cup | 20.7 |
| Cucumber, peeled, raw | 1 large | 20.2 |
| Vegetables, mixed, canned, drained solids | 1 cup | 20.2 |
| Beans, snap, green, cooked, boiled, drained, without salt | 1 cup | 20.0 |
| Beans, snap, yellow, cooked, boiled, drained, without salt | 1 cup | 20.0 |
| Carrots, frozen, cooked, boiled, drained, without salt | 1 cup | 19.9 |
| Soup, vegetable, canned, chunky, ready-to-serve, | 1 cup | 19.4 |

# Vitamin K Levels in Common Foods

| | | |
|---|---|---|
| commercial | | |
| Fast foods, potato, french fried in vegetable oil | 1 large | 18.9 |
| Salad dressing, french dressing, commercial, regular | 1 tbsp | 18.9 |
| Artichokes, (globe or french), cooked, boiled, drained, without salt | 1 medium | 17.8 |
| Spices, parsley, dried | 1 tbsp | 17.7 |
| Eclairs, custard-filled with chocolate glaze, prepared from recipe | 1 eclair | 17.5 |
| Lettuce, green leaf, raw | 1 leaf | 17.4 |
| Beans, snap, green, frozen, cooked, boiled, drained without salt | 1 cup | 17.1 |
| Beans, snap, yellow, frozen, cooked, boiled, drained, without salt | 1 cup | 17.1 |
| Cauliflower, cooked, boiled, drained, without salt | 1 cup | 17.1 |
| Cucumber, with peel, raw | 1 cup | 17.1 |
| Vegetable oil, canola | 1 tbsp | 17.1 |
| Raspberries, frozen, red, sweetened | 1 cup | 16.3 |
| Cauliflower, raw | 1 cup | 16.0 |
| Candies, white chocolate | 1 cup | 15.5 |
| Fast Foods, biscuit, with egg and sausage | 1 biscuit | 15.5 |
| Salad dressing, home recipe, vinegar and oil | 1 tbsp | 15.4 |
| Nuts, pine nuts, dried | 1 oz | 15.3 |
| Fast foods, potato, french fried in vegetable oil | 1 medium | 15.0 |

| | | |
|---|---|---|
| Margarine-butter blend, 60% corn oil margarine and 40% butter | 1 tbsp | 14.7 |
| Carrots, raw | 1 cup | 14.5 |
| Margarine, vegetable oil spread, 60% fat, stick | 1 tbsp | 14.5 |
| Carrots, canned, regular pack, drained solids | 1 cup | 14.3 |
| Celery, cooked, boiled, drained, without salt | 1 stalk | 14.2 |
| Tomatoes, red, ripe, raw, year round average | 1 cup | 14.2 |
| Salad dressing, blue or roquefort cheese dressing, commercial, regular | 1 tbsp | 13.9 |
| Bread stuffing, bread, dry mix, prepared | 1/2 cup | 13.7 |
| Beans, snap, green, canned, regular pack, drained solids | 1 cup | 13.4 |
| Beans, snap, yellow, canned, regular pack, drained solids | 1 cup | 13.4 |
| Seeds, pumpkin and squash seed kernels, roasted, with salt added | 1 oz (142 seeds) | 13.4 |
| Turkey patties, breaded, battered, fried | 1 patty | 13.4 |
| Lettuce, iceberg (includes crisphead types), raw | 1 cup | 13.3 |
| Margarine, regular, tub, composite, 80% fat, with salt | 1 tbsp | 13.2 |
| Margarine, regular, unspecified oils, with salt added | 1 tbsp | 13.1 |
| Peppers, sweet, green, | 1 cup | 12.9 |

| | | |
|---|---|---|
| cooked, boiled, drained, without salt | | |
| Vegetable juice cocktail, canned | 1 cup | 12.8 |
| Potatoes, mashed, home-prepared, whole milk and margarine added | 1 cup | 12.6 |
| Pickle relish, sweet | 1 tbsp | 12.5 |
| Pears, asian, raw | 1 pear | 12.4 |
| Pie, blueberry, commercially prepared | 1 piece | 12.3 |
| Pickles, cucumber, dill | 1 pickle | 11.9 |
| Celery, raw | 1 stalk | 11.7 |
| Nuts, chestnuts, european, roasted | 1 cup | 11.2 |
| Plums, canned, purple, heavy syrup pack, solids and liquids | 1 cup | 11.1 |
| Peppers, sweet, green, raw | 1 cup | 11.0 |
| Plums, canned, purple, juice pack, solids and liquids | 1 cup | 10.8 |
| Salad dressing, thousand island, commercial, regular | 1 tbsp | 10.8 |
| Fast foods, french toast sticks | 5 sticks | 10.6 |
| Lettuce, cos or romaine, raw | 1 leaf | 10.3 |
| Pie crust, standard-type, frozen, ready-to-bake, baked | 1 pie shell | 10.3 |
| Snacks, corn-based, extruded, puffs or twists, cheese-flavor | 1 oz | 10.2 |
| Alfalfa seeds, sprouted, raw | 1 cup | 10.1 |
| Nuts, cashew nuts, dry roasted, with salt added | 1 oz | 9.8 |
| Nuts, cashew nuts, oil | 1 oz (18 | 9.8 |

| | | |
|---|---|---|
| roasted, with salt added | nuts) | |
| Peas, split, mature seeds, cooked, boiled, without salt | 1 cup | 9.8 |
| Tomatoes, red, ripe, raw, year round average | 1 tomato | 9.7 |
| Raspberries, raw | 1 cup | 9.6 |
| Carrots, raw | 1 carrot | 9.5 |
| Fast foods, potato, french fried in vegetable oil | 1 small | 9.5 |
| Candies, semisweet chocolate | 1 cup | 9.4 |
| Lima beans, immature seeds, frozen, baby, cooked, boiled, drained, without salt | 1 cup | 9.4 |
| Spices, oregano, dried | 1 tsp | 9.3 |
| Squash, winter, all varieties, cooked, baked, without salt | 1 cup | 9.0 |
| Pie, cherry, commercially prepared | 1 piece | 8.9 |
| Peppers, sweet, green, raw | 1 pepper | 8.8 |
| Lima beans, immature seeds, frozen, fordhook, cooked, boiled, drained, without salt | 1 cup | 8.7 |
| Mangos, raw | 1 mango | 8.7 |
| Prune juice, canned | 1 cup | 8.7 |
| Cucumber, peeled, raw | 1 cup | 8.6 |
| Tomato products, canned, puree, without salt added | 1 cup | 8.5 |
| Buckwheat flour, whole-groat | 1 cup | 8.4 |
| Duck, domesticated, meat only, cooked, roasted | 1/2 duck | 8.4 |
| Salad dressing, italian dressing, commercial, regular | 1 tbsp | 8.2 |

Vitamin K Levels in Common Foods

| Salad dressing, russian dressing | 1 tbsp | 8.2 |
|---|---|---|
| Beef stew, canned entree | 1 cup | 8.1 |
| Oil, olive, salad or cooking | 1 tbsp | 8.1 |
| Papayas, raw | 1 papaya | 7.9 |
| Lettuce, butterhead (includes boston and bibb types), raw | 1 medium leaf | 7.7 |
| Cauliflower, cooked, boiled, drained, without salt | 3 flowerets | 7.5 |
| Cereals, oats, regular and quick and instant, unenriched, cooked with water, without salt | 1 cup | 7.5 |
| Pears, raw | 1 pear | 7.5 |
| Fast foods, chicken, breaded and fried, boneless pieces, plain | 6 pieces | 7.4 |
| Muffins, oat bran | 1 muffin | 7.4 |
| Soy milk, fluid | 1 cup | 7.4 |
| Grapes, red or green (european type varieties, such as, Thompson seedless), raw | 10 grapes | 7.3 |
| Peppers, sweet, red, raw | 1 cup | 7.3 |
| Soup, pea, green, canned, prepared with equal volume water, commercial | 1 cup | 7.3 |
| Soup, clam chowder, manhattan, canned, prepared with equal volume water | 1 cup | 7.1 |
| Mangos, raw | 1 cup | 6.9 |
| Peppers, sweet, red, cooked, boiled, drained, without salt | 1 cup | 6.9 |

| | | |
|---|---|---|
| Tomato products, canned, sauce | 1 cup | 6.9 |
| Fast Food, Pizza Chain, 14" pizza, pepperoni topping, regular crust | 1 slice | 6.8 |
| Pie, pumpkin, commercially prepared | 1 piece | 6.8 |
| Tomatoes, red, ripe, canned, whole, regular pack | 1 cup | 6.7 |
| Chickpeas (garbanzo beans, bengal gram), mature seeds, cooked, boiled, without salt | 1 cup | 6.6 |
| Seaweed, kelp, raw | 2 tbsp | 6.6 |
| Chives, raw | 1 tbsp | 6.4 |
| Fruit cocktail, (peach and pineapple and pear and grape and cherry), canned, heavy syrup, solids and liquids | 1 cup | 6.4 |
| Peppers, hot chili, green, raw | 1 pepper | 6.4 |
| Peppers, hot chili, red, raw | 1 pepper | 6.3 |
| Snacks, potato chips, plain, salted | 1 oz | 6.3 |
| Snacks, potato chips, plain, unsalted | 1 oz | 6.3 |
| Soup, vegetarian vegetable, canned, prepared with equal volume water, commercial | 1 cup | 6.3 |
| Squash, summer, all varieties, cooked, boiled, drained, without salt | 1 cup | 6.3 |
| Fruit cocktail, (peach and pineapple and pear and grape and cherry), canned, juice pack, solids and liquids | 1 cup | 6.2 |

| | | |
|---|---|---|
| Fish, fish portions and sticks, frozen, preheated | 1 portion (4" x 2" x 1/2") | 6.1 |
| Peaches, dried, sulfured, uncooked | 3 halves | 6.1 |
| Tomatoes, red, ripe, canned, stewed | 1 cup | 6.1 |
| Avocados, raw, California | 1 oz | 6.0 |
| Beans, pinto, mature seeds, cooked, boiled, without salt | 1 cup | 6.0 |
| Refried beans, canned (includes USDA commodity) | 1 cup | 6.0 |
| Veal, leg (top round), separable lean and fat, cooked, braised | 3 oz | 6.0 |
| Figs, dried, uncooked | 2 figs | 5.9 |
| Muffins, wheat bran, toaster-type with raisins, toasted | 1 muffin | 5.9 |
| Beans, kidney, red, mature seeds, cooked, boiled, without salt | 1 cup | 5.8 |
| Doughnuts, yeast-leavened, glazed, enriched (includes honey buns) | 1 medium | 5.8 |
| Peppers, sweet, red, raw | 1 pepper | 5.8 |
| Potatoes, hashed brown, home-prepared | 1 cup | 5.8 |
| Salad dressing, mayonnaise, soybean oil, with salt | 1 tbsp | 5.8 |
| Apricots, canned, heavy syrup pack, with skin, solids and liquids | 1 cup | 5.7 |
| Beans, kidney, red, mature seeds, canned | 1 cup | 5.6 |
| Sweet potato, canned, | 1 cup | 5.6 |

| | | |
|---|---|---|
| vacuum pack | | |
| Tomato juice, canned, with salt added | 1 cup | 5.6 |
| Turkey, all classes, neck, meat only, cooked, simmered | 1 neck | 5.6 |
| Peaches, frozen, sliced, sweetened | 1 cup | 5.5 |
| Pears, asian, raw | 1 pear | 5.5 |
| Shortening, household, soybean (hydrogenated)-cottonseed (hydrogenated) | 1 tbsp | 5.5 |
| Apricots, canned, juice pack, with skin, solids and liquids | 1 cup | 5.4 |
| Pie, pecan, commercially prepared | 1 piece | 5.4 |
| Danish pastry, cheese | 1 danish | 5.3 |
| Pie, fried pies, fruit | 1 pie | 5.2 |
| Snacks, fruit leather, pieces | 1 oz | 5.2 |
| Turkey, all classes, meat only, cooked, roasted | 1 cup | 5.2 |
| Fast foods, chili con carne | 1 cup | 5.1 |
| Raisins, seedless | 1 cup | 5.1 |
| Sweet potato, canned, syrup pack, drained solids | 1 cup | 5.1 |
| Shake, fast food, chocolate | 16 fl oz | 5.0 |
| Frostings, vanilla, creamy, ready-to-eat | 1/12 package | 4.9 |
| Margarine, vegetable oil spread, 60% fat, stick | 1 tsp | 4.9 |
| Margarine, vegetable oil spread, 60% fat, tub/bottle | 1 tsp | 4.9 |
| Melons, honeydew, raw | 1 cup | 4.9 |
| Dates, deglet noor | 1 cup | 4.8 |
| HEALTHY CHOICE Beef | 1 package | 4.8 |

| | | |
|---|---|---|
| Macaroni, frozen entree | | |
| Cake, white, prepared from recipe with coconut frosting | 1 piece | 4.6 |
| Melons, honeydew, raw | 1/8 melon | 4.6 |
| Nuts, pine nuts, dried | 1 tbsp | 4.6 |
| Margarine-like spread, (approximately 40% fat), unspecified oils | 1 tsp | 4.5 |
| Pasta with meatballs in tomato sauce, canned entree | 1 cup | 4.5 |
| Peaches, canned, heavy syrup pack, solids and liquids | 1 cup | 4.5 |
| Barley, pearled, raw | 1 cup | 4.4 |
| Peaches, raw | 1 cup | 4.4 |
| Snacks, popcorn, caramel-coated, without peanuts | 1 cup | 4.4 |
| Soup, vegetable beef, prepared with equal volume water, commercial | 1 cup | 4.4 |
| Chicken, stewing, meat only, cooked, stewed | 1 cup | 4.3 |
| Strawberries, frozen, sweetened, sliced | 1 cup | 4.3 |
| Peaches, canned, juice pack, solids and liquids | 1 cup | 4.2 |
| Pizza, cheese topping, regular crust, frozen, cooked | 1 serving | 4.2 |
| Plums, raw | 1 plum | 4.2 |
| Salad dressing, thousand island dressing, reduced fat | 1 tbsp | 4.2 |
| Lamb, domestic, loin, separable lean and fat, trimmed to 1/4" fat, choice, | 3 oz | 4.1 |

| | | |
|---|---|---|
| cooked, broiled | | |
| Pie, apple, commercially prepared, enriched flour | 1 piece | 4.1 |
| Melons, cantaloupe, raw | 1 cup | 4.0 |
| Nuts, hazelnuts or filberts | 1 oz | 4.0 |
| Potato, baked, flesh and skin, without salt | 1 potato | 4.0 |
| Cookies, graham crackers, plain or honey (includes cinnamon) | 1 cup | 3.9 |
| Soup, tomato, canned, prepared with equal volume water, commercial | 1 cup | 3.9 |
| Cake, white, prepared from recipe without frosting | 1 piece | 3.8 |
| Danish pastry, fruit, enriched (includes apple, cinnamon, raisin, lemon, raspberry, strawberry) | 1 danish | 3.8 |
| Lima beans, large, mature seeds, cooked, boiled, without salt | 1 cup | 3.8 |
| Potatoes, mashed, home-prepared, whole milk added | 1 cup | 3.8 |
| Snacks, fruit leather, rolls | 1 large | 3.8 |
| Snacks, potato chips, reduced fat | 1 oz | 3.8 |
| Soup, chicken noodle, canned, chunky, ready-to-serve | 1 cup | 3.8 |
| Nuts, mixed nuts, dry roasted, with peanuts, with salt added | 1 oz | 3.7 |
| Nuts, pistachio nuts, dry roasted, with salt added | 1 oz (47 nuts) | 3.7 |

# Vitamin K Levels in Common Foods

| | | |
|---|---|---|
| Strawberries, raw | 1 cup | 3.7 |
| Cookies, brownies, commercially prepared | 1 brownie | 3.6 |
| Cookies, sugar, prepared from recipe, made with margarine | 1 cookie | 3.6 |
| Lamb, domestic, leg, whole (shank and sirloin), separable lean and fat, trimmed to 1/4" fat, choice, cooked, roasted | 3 oz | 3.6 |
| Nuts, mixed nuts, oil roasted, with peanuts, with salt added | 1 oz | 3.6 |
| Papayas, raw | 1 cup | 3.6 |
| Soup, chicken noodle, dehydrated, prepared with water | 1 cup | 3.5 |
| Cherries, sour, red, canned, water pack, solids and liquids (includes USDA commodity red tart cherries, canned) | 1 cup | 3.4 |
| Chicken, broilers or fryers, breast, meat and skin, cooked, fried, batter | 1/2 breast | 3.4 |
| Lentils, mature seeds, cooked, boiled, without salt | 1 cup | 3.4 |
| Oil, soybean, salad or cooking, (hydrogenated) | 1 tbsp | 3.4 |
| Oil, soybean, salad or cooking, (hydrogenated) and cottonseed | 1 tbsp | 3.4 |
| Peppers, jalapeno, canned, solids and liquids | 1/4 cup | 3.4 |
| Spices, pepper, black | 1 tsp | 3.4 |
| Squash, summer, all | 1 cup | 3.4 |

| | | |
|---|---|---|
| varieties, raw | | |
| Sweet potato, cooked, baked in skin, without salt | 1 potato | 3.4 |
| Beef, variety meats and by-products, liver, cooked, pan-fried | 3 oz | 3.3 |
| Lamb, domestic, loin, separable lean only, trimmed to 1/4" fat, choice, cooked, broiled | 3 oz | 3.3 |
| Potatoes, boiled, cooked without skin, flesh, without salt | 1 cup | 3.3 |
| Sweet potato, cooked, boiled, without skin | 1 potato | 3.3 |
| Tomatillos, raw | 1 medium | 3.3 |
| Turkey, all classes, dark meat, cooked, roasted | 3 oz | 3.3 |
| Buckwheat groats, roasted, cooked | 1 cup | 3.2 |
| Potato puffs, frozen, oven-heated | 10 puffs | 3.2 |
| Potatoes, mashed, dehydrated, prepared from flakes without milk, whole milk and butter added | 1 cup | 3.2 |
| Lamb, domestic, leg, whole (shank and sirloin), separable lean only, trimmed to 1/4" fat, choice, cooked, roasted | 3 oz | 3.1 |
| Muffins, blueberry, commercially prepared | 1 muffin | 3.1 |
| Apples, raw, with skin | 1 apple | 3.0 |
| Croutons, seasoned | 1 cup | 3.0 |

| | | |
|---|---|---|
| Fish, fish portions and sticks, frozen, preheated | 1 stick (4" x 1" x 1/2") | 3.0 |
| Grape juice, frozen concentrate, sweetened, undiluted, with added vitamin C | 6-fl-oz can | 3.0 |
| Nectarines, raw | 1 nectarine | 3.0 |
| Noodles, chinese, chow mein | 1 cup | 3.0 |
| Oat bran, raw | 1 cup | 3.0 |
| Soup, bean with pork, canned, prepared with equal volume water, commercial | 1 cup | 3.0 |
| Cake, boston cream pie, commercially prepared | 1 piece | 2.9 |
| Cookies, chocolate sandwich, with creme filling, regular | 1 cookie | 2.9 |
| Cowpeas, common (blackeyes, crowder, southern), mature seeds, cooked, boiled, without salt | 1 cup | 2.9 |
| Eggplant, cooked, boiled, drained, without salt | 1 cup | 2.9 |
| Potatoes, boiled, cooked in skin, flesh, without salt | 1 potato | 2.9 |
| Potatoes, boiled, cooked without skin, flesh, without salt | 1 potato | 2.8 |
| Baking chocolate, unsweetened, squares | 1 square | 2.7 |
| Bulgur, dry | 1 cup | 2.7 |
| Cheese, ricotta, whole milk | 1 cup | 2.7 |

| | | |
|---|---|---|
| Soup, cream of mushroom, canned, prepared with equal volume milk, commercial | 1 cup | 2.7 |
| Spices, chili powder | 1 tsp | 2.7 |
| Beans, baked, canned, with franks | 1 cup | 2.6 |
| Chicken, canned, meat only, with broth | 5 oz | 2.6 |
| Egg, whole, cooked, fried | 1 large | 2.6 |
| Sweet rolls, cinnamon, commercially prepared with raisins | 1 roll | 2.6 |
| Candies, milk chocolate | 1 bar (1.55 oz) | 2.5 |
| Cranberry juice cocktail, bottled | 8 fl oz | 2.5 |
| Doughnuts, cake-type, plain (includes unsugared, old-fashioned) | 1 medium | 2.5 |
| Peaches, raw | 1 peach | 2.5 |
| Soup, tomato, canned, prepared with equal volume milk, commercial | 1 cup | 2.5 |
| Egg, whole, cooked, scrambled | 1 large | 2.4 |
| Pie, lemon meringue, commercially prepared | 1 piece | 2.4 |
| Tofu, soft, prepared with calcium sulfate and magnesium chloride (nigari) | 1 piece | 2.4 |
| Candies, M&M MARS, MARS MILKY WAY Bar | 1 bar (2.15 oz) | 2.3 |
| Candies, REESE'S Peanut Butter Cups | 1 package (contains 2) | 2.3 |

| | | |
|---|---|---|
| Pancakes plain, frozen, ready-to-heat (includes buttermilk) | 1 pancake | 2.3 |
| Sauce, homemade, white, medium | 1 cup | 2.3 |
| Wheat flour, whole-grain | 1 cup | 2.3 |
| Candies, carob | 1 oz | 2.2 |
| Candies, KIT KAT Wafer Bar | 1 bar (1.5 oz) | 2.2 |
| Fish, sardine, Atlantic, canned in oil, drained solids with bone | 3 oz | 2.2 |
| Salad dressing, home recipe, cooked | 1 tbsp | 2.2 |
| Soup, clam chowder, new england, canned, prepared with equal volume milk, commercial | 1 cup | 2.2 |
| Waffles, plain, frozen, ready -to-heat, toasted | 1 waffle | 2.2 |
| Candies, milk chocolate, with almonds | 1 bar (1.45 oz) | 2.1 |
| Cauliflower, raw | 1 floweret | 2.1 |
| Cereals ready-to-eat, QUAKER, QUAKER 100% Natural Cereal with oats, honey, and raisins | 1/2 cup | 2.1 |
| Chocolate-flavor beverage mix for milk, powder, without added nutrients | 2-3 heaping tsp | 2.1 |
| Fish, tuna, white, canned in water, drained solids | 3 oz | 2.1 |
| Potato pancakes | 1 pancake | 2.1 |
| Toaster pastries, fruit (includes apple, blueberry, | 1 pastry | 2.1 |

| | | |
|---|---|---|
| cherry, strawberry) | | |
| Beans, baked, canned, plain or vegetarian | 1 cup | 2.0 |
| Beans, baked, canned, with pork and sweet sauce | 1 cup | 2.0 |
| Chicken, broilers or fryers, thigh, meat only, cooked, roasted | 1 thigh | 2.0 |
| Cookies, oatmeal, commercially prepared, regular | 1 cookie | 2.0 |
| Plums, canned, purple, heavy syrup pack, solids and liquids | 1 plum | 2.0 |
| Plums, canned, purple, juice pack, solids and liquids | 1 plum | 2.0 |
| Pumpkin, cooked, boiled, drained, without salt | 1 cup | 2.0 |
| Snacks, potato chips, made from dried potatoes, light | 1 oz | 2.0 |
| Snacks, potato chips, made from dried potatoes, plain | 1 oz | 2.0 |
| Soup, cream of mushroom, canned, prepared with equal volume water, commercial | 1 cup | 2.0 |
| Spaghetti with meat sauce, frozen entree | 1 package | 2.0 |
| Spices, curry powder | 1 tsp | 2.0 |
| Beef, ground, 75% lean meat / 25% fat, patty, cooked, broiled | 3 oz | 1.9 |
| Bread crumbs, dry, grated, plain | 1 oz | 1.9 |
| Cereals ready-to-eat, GENERAL MILLS, | 3/4 cup | 1.9 |

| | | |
|---|---|---|
| CINNAMON TOAST CRUNCH | | |
| Lettuce, iceberg (includes crisphead types), raw | 1 medium | 1.9 |
| Salad dressing, italian dressing, reduced fat | 1 tbsp | 1.9 |
| Candies, MR. GOODBAR Chocolate Bar | 1 bar (1.75 oz) | 1.8 |
| Cookies, molasses | 1 cookie, large (3-1/2" to 4" | 1.8 |
| Milk, canned, condensed, sweetened | 1 cup | 1.8 |
| Oil, sesame, salad or cooking | 1 tbsp | 1.8 |
| Snacks, corn-based, extruded, chips, plain | 1 oz | 1.8 |
| Cheese, ricotta, part skim milk | 1 cup | 1.7 |
| Melons, cantaloupe, raw | 1/8 melon | 1.7 |
| Peaches, canned, heavy syrup pack, solids and liquids | 1 half | 1.7 |
| Peaches, canned, juice pack, solids and liquids | 1 half | 1.7 |
| Snacks, popcorn, oil-popped, microwaved | 1 cup | 1.7 |
| Spices, paprika | 1 tsp | 1.7 |
| Beef, round, eye of round, separable lean only, trimmed to 1/8" fat, all grades, cooked, roasted | 3 oz | 1.6 |
| Candies, milk chocolate coated peanuts | 10 pieces | 1.6 |
| Cereals ready-to-eat, | 1/2 cup | 1.6 |

| KELLOGG, KELLOGG'S ALLBRAN Original | | |
|---|---|---|
| Parsnips, cooked, boiled, drained, without salt | 1 cup | 1.6 |
| Snacks, popcorn, caramel-coated, with peanuts | 1 cup | 1.6 |
| Tomatoes, red, ripe, raw, year round average | 1 slice | 1.6 |
| Applesauce, canned, sweetened, without salt | 1 cup | 1.5 |
| Applesauce, canned, unsweetened, without added ascorbic acid | 1 cup | 1.5 |
| Cereals ready-to-eat, GENERAL MILLS, BASIC 4 | 1 cup | 1.5 |
| Cereals ready-to-eat, QUAKER, Low Fat 100% Natural Granola with Raisins | 1/2 cup | 1.5 |
| Chicken, broilers or fryers, drumstick, meat only, cooked, roasted | 1 drumstick | 1.5 |
| Cookies, sugar, refrigerated dough, baked | 1 cookie | 1.5 |
| Beef, chuck, blade roast, separable lean only, trimmed to 1/4" fat, all grades, cooked, braised | 3 oz | 1.4 |
| Beef, cured, corned beef, canned | 3 oz | 1.4 |
| Beef, ground, 80% lean meat / 20% fat, patty, cooked, broiled | 3 oz | 1.4 |
| Beef, round, bottom round, separable lean and fat, trimmed to 1/8" fat, all grades, cooked, braised | 3 oz | 1.4 |

| Food | Serving | Amount |
|---|---|---|
| Beef, round, bottom round, separable lean only, trimmed to 1/8" fat, all grades, cooked, braised | 3 oz | 1.4 |
| Beef, top sirloin, separable lean and fat, trimmed to 1/8" fat, all grades, cooked, broiled | 3 oz | 1.4 |
| Bread, white, commercially prepared (includes soft bread crumbs) | 1 cup | 1.4 |
| Cake, snack cakes, creme-filled, chocolate with frosting | 1 cupcake | 1.4 |
| Cherries, sweet, raw | 10 cherries | 1.4 |
| Barley, pearled, cooked | 1 cup | 1.3 |
| Beans, baked, canned, with pork and tomato sauce | 1 cup | 1.3 |
| Bread, Indian, fry, made with lard (Navajo) | 10-1/2" bread | 1.3 |
| Cocoa mix, with aspartame, powder, prepared from item 14196 | 1 serving | 1.3 |
| Cookies, sugar, commercially prepared, regular (includes vanilla) | 1 cookie | 1.3 |
| Crackers, whole-wheat | 4 crackers | 1.3 |
| Milk, canned, evaporated, without added vitamin A | 1 cup | 1.3 |
| Muffins, corn, commercially prepared | 1 muffin | 1.3 |
| Plantains, raw | 1 medium | 1.3 |
| Potatoes, french fried, all types, salt added in processing, frozen, home prepared, oven heated | 10 strips | 1.3 |

| | | |
|---|---|---|
| Rolls, hamburger or hotdog, plain | 1 roll | 1.3 |
| Shake, fast food, vanilla | 16 fl oz | 1.3 |
| Tomatoes, red, ripe, raw, year round average | 1 cherry tomato | 1.3 |
| Apricots, raw | 1 apricot | 1.2 |
| Beef, round, eye of round, separable lean and fat, trimmed to 1/8" fat, all grades, cooked, roasted | 3 oz | 1.2 |
| Beef, top sirloin, separable lean only, trimmed to 1/8" fat, all grades, cooked, broiled | 3 oz | 1.2 |
| Cereals ready-to-eat, GENERAL MILLS, RAISIN NUT BRAN | 1 cup | 1.2 |
| Doughnuts, yeast-leavened, glazed, enriched (includes honey buns) | 1 hole | 1.2 |
| Lime juice, canned or bottled, unsweetened | 1 cup | 1.2 |
| Rice, brown, long-grain, cooked | 1 cup | 1.2 |
| Soup, beef noodle, canned, prepared with equal volume water, commercial | 1 cup | 1.2 |
| Apricots, dried, sulfured, uncooked | 10 halves | 1.1 |
| Beans, navy, mature seeds, cooked, boiled, without salt | 1 cup | 1.1 |
| Candies, M&M MARS, SNICKERS Bar | 1 bar (2 oz) | 1.1 |
| Cookies, chocolate chip, commercially prepared, reg, higher fat, enriched | 1 cookie | 1.1 |

| | | |
|---|---|---|
| Dates, deglet noor | 5 dates | 1.1 |
| Malted drink mix, natural, with added nutrients, powder, prepared with whole milk | 1 cup | 1.1 |
| Onions, cooked, boiled, drained, without salt | 1 cup | 1.1 |
| Pineapple, raw, all varieties | 1 cup | 1.1 |
| Plantains, cooked | 1 cup | 1.1 |
| Potatoes, hashed brown, frozen, plain, prepared | 1 patty | 1.1 |
| Puddings, chocolate, ready-to-eat | 4 oz | 1.1 |
| Salad dressing, russian dressing, low calorie | 1 tbsp | 1.1 |
| Tortillas, ready-to-bake or -fry, flour | 1 tortilla | 1.1 |
| Apples, dried, sulfured, uncooked | 5 rings | 1.0 |
| Bagels, plain, enriched, with calcium propionate (includes onion, poppy, sesame) | 4" bagel | 1.0 |
| Beef, ground, 85% lean meat / 15% fat, patty, cooked, broiled | 3 oz | 1.0 |
| Butter, salted | 1 tbsp | 1.0 |
| Butter, without salt | 1 tbsp | 1.0 |
| Cereals ready-to-eat, KELLOGG, KELLOGG'S RAISIN BRAN | 1 cup | 1.0 |
| Cheese food, pasteurized process, american, without di sodium phosphate | 1 oz | 1.0 |
| Crackers, saltines (includes oyster, soda, soup) | 4 crackers | 1.0 |

| | | |
|---|---|---|
| Croissants, butter | 1 croissant | 1.0 |
| Grape juice, canned or bottled, unsweetened, without added vitamin C | 1 cup | 1.0 |
| Grape juice, frozen concentrate, sweetened, diluted with 3 volume water, with added vitamin C | 1 cup | 1.0 |
| Ice creams, vanilla, rich | 1/2 cup | 1.0 |
| Nuts, pecans | 1 oz (20 halves) | 1.0 |
| Oil, vegetable safflower, salad or cooking, oleic, over 70% (primary safflower oil of commerce) | 1 tbsp | 1.0 |
| Pimento, canned | 1 tbsp | 1.0 |
| Potatoes, baked, skin, without salt | 1 skin | 1.0 |
| Puddings, tapioca, ready-to-eat | 4 oz | 1.0 |
| Spaghetti, whole-wheat, cooked | 1 cup | 1.0 |
| Spinach souffle | 136 | 1 cup |
| Spinach, canned, drained solids | 214 | 1 cup |
| Braunschweiger (a liver sausage), pork | 2 slices | 0.9 |
| Bulgur, cooked | 1 cup | 0.9 |
| Carrots, baby, raw | 1 medium | 0.9 |
| Cereals ready-to-eat, GENERAL MILLS, TOTAL Raisin Bran | 1 cup | 0.9 |
| Cereals, oats, instant, fortified, plain, prepared with | 1 packet | 0.9 |

| | | |
|---|---|---|
| water | | |
| Cheese, cottage, creamed, with fruit | 1 cup | 0.9 |
| Cookies, fig bars | 1 cookie | 0.9 |
| Fish, roughy, orange, cooked, dry heat | 3 oz | 0.9 |
| Orange juice, frozen concentrate, unsweetened, undiluted | 6-fl-oz can | 0.9 |
| Seeds, sunflower seed kernels, dry roasted, with salt added | 1/4 cup | 0.9 |
| Tomatoes, sun-dried | 1 piece | 0.9 |
| Turkey, all classes, giblets, cooked, simmered, some giblet fat | 1 cup | 0.9 |
| Bagels, plain, enriched, with calcium propionate (includes onion, poppy, sesame) | 3-1/2" bagel | 0.8 |
| Bananas, raw | 1 cup | 0.8 |
| Bread, white, commercially prepared (includes soft bread crumbs) | 1 slice | 0.8 |
| Cereals ready-to-eat, KELLOGG, KELLOGG'S FROSTED MINI WHEATS, bite size | 1 cup | 0.8 |
| Cereals ready-to-eat, KELLOGG'S FROSTED MINIWHEATS, original | 1 cup | 0.8 |
| Cereals, QUAKER, Instant Oatmeal, maple and brown sugar, prepared with boiling water | 1 packet | 0.8 |
| Cheese, camembert | 1 wedge | 0.8 |

| Cheese, cheddar | 1 oz | 0.8 |
|---|---|---|
| Cheese, cottage, creamed, large or small curd | 1 cup | 0.8 |
| Cheese, pasteurized process, american, with di sodium phosphate | 1 oz | 0.8 |
| Chocolate-flavor beverage mix, powder, prepared with whole milk | 1 cup | 0.8 |
| Cookies, molasses | 1 cookie, medium | 0.8 |
| Cookies, shortbread, commercially prepared, plain | 1 cookie | 0.8 |
| Cookies, vanilla sandwich with creme filling | 1 cookie | 0.8 |
| Crackers, cheese, sandwich-type with peanut butter filling | 1 sandwich | 0.8 |
| Crackers, standard snack-type, regular | 4 crackers | 0.8 |
| Crackers, wheat, regular | 4 crackers | 0.8 |
| Cranberry sauce, canned, sweetened | 1 slice | 0.8 |
| Doughnuts, cake-type, plain (includes unsugared, old-fashioned) | 1 hole | 0.8 |
| Frankfurter, beef | 1 frank | 0.8 |
| Frankfurter, beef and pork | 1 frank | 0.8 |
| Ice creams, french vanilla, soft-serve | 1/2 cup | 0.8 |
| Malted drink mix, chocolate, with added nutrients, powder, prepared with whole milk | 1 cup | 0.8 |
| Nuts, walnuts, english | 1 oz (14 halves) | 0.8 |

| | | |
|---|---|---|
| Pears, canned, heavy syrup pack, solids and liquids | 1 cup | 0.8 |
| Pineapple juice, canned, unsweetened, without added ascorbic acid | 1 cup | 0.8 |
| Pineapple, canned, heavy syrup pack, solids and liquids | 1 cup | 0.8 |
| Rolls, dinner, plain, commercially prepared (includes brown-and-serve) | 1 roll | 0.8 |
| Salad dressing, french dressing, reduced fat | 1 tbsp | 0.8 |
| Seeds, sunflower seed kernels, dry roasted, with salt added | 1 oz | 0.8 |
| Wild rice, cooked | 1 cup | 0.8 |
| Apples, raw, without skin | 1 cup | 0.7 |
| Bread, Indian, fry, made with lard (Navajo) | 5" bread | 0.7 |
| Bread, white, commercially prepared, toasted | 1 slice | 0.7 |
| Candies, caramels, chocolate-flavor roll | 1 piece | 0.7 |
| Candies, M&M MARS, MARS MILKY WAY Bar | 1 fun size bar | 0.7 |
| Cereals, QUAKER,Instant Oatmeal, apples and cinnamon, prepared with boiling water | 1 packet | 0.7 |
| Cheese, blue | 1 oz | 0.7 |
| Cheese, mozzarella, whole milk | 1 oz | 0.7 |
| Cheese, muenster | 1 oz | 0.7 |
| Cheese, swiss | 1 oz | 0.7 |

| | | |
|---|---|---|
| Cookies, peanut butter, commercially prepared, regular | 1 cookie | 0.7 |
| English muffins, plain, enriched, with ca prop (includes sourdough) | 1 muffin | 0.7 |
| English muffins, plain, toasted, enriched, with calcium propionate (includes sourdough) | 1 muffin | 0.7 |
| Fast foods, ice milk, vanilla, soft-serve, with cone | 1 cone | 0.7 |
| Frozen novelties, fruit and juice bars | 1 bar (2.5 fl oz) | 0.7 |
| Oil, vegetable, sunflower, linoleic, (approx. 65%) | 1 tbsp | 0.7 |
| Pears, canned, juice pack, solids and liquids | 1 cup | 0.7 |
| Peppers, sweet, green, raw | 1 ring | 0.7 |
| Pineapple, canned, juice pack, solids and liquids | 1 cup | 0.7 |
| Poultry food products, ground turkey, cooked | 1 patty | 0.7 |
| Salami, cooked, beef and pork | 2 slices | 0.7 |
| Sauce, ready-to-serve, salsa | 1 tbsp | 0.7 |
| Snacks, oriental mix, rice-based | 1 oz (about 1/4 cup) | 0.7 |
| Spices, cinnamon, ground | 1 tsp | 0.7 |
| Taco shells, baked | 1 medium | 0.7 |
| Bagels, cinnamon-raisin | 4" bagel | 0.6 |
| Bananas, raw | 1 banana | 0.6 |
| Biscuits, plain or buttermilk, refrigerated dough, higher | 2-1/2" biscuit | 0.6 |

| | | |
|---|---|---|
| fat, baked | | |
| Bread, mixed-grain (includes whole-grain, 7-grain) | 1 slice | 0.6 |
| Bread, whole-wheat, commercially prepared | 1 slice | 0.6 |
| Bread, whole-wheat, commercially prepared, toasted | 1 slice | 0.6 |
| Cake, fruitcake, commercially prepared | 1 piece | 0.6 |
| Cake, snack cakes, creme-filled, sponge | 1 cake | 0.6 |
| Candies, M&M MARS, "M&M's" Peanut Chocolate Candies | 10 pieces | 0.6 |
| Cereals ready-to-eat, QUAKER, Honey Nut Heaven | 1 cup | 0.6 |
| Cereals ready-to-eat, wheat, shredded, plain, sugar and salt free | 2 biscuits | 0.6 |
| Cheese, pasteurized process, swiss, with di sodium phosphate | 1 oz | 0.6 |
| Cheese, provolone | 1 oz | 0.6 |
| Cookies, graham crackers, plain or honey (includes cinnamon) | 2 squares | 0.6 |
| Crackers, rye, wafers, plain | 1 wafer | 0.6 |
| Crackers, standard snack-type, sandwich, with cheese filling | 1 sandwich | 0.6 |
| Malted drink mix, chocolate, with added nutrients, powder | 3 heaping tsp | 0.6 |
| Milk shakes, thick chocolate | 10.6 fl oz | 0.6 |

| | | |
|---|---|---|
| Milk shakes, thick vanilla | 11 fl oz | 0.6 |
| Onions, raw | 1 cup | 0.6 |
| Turkey roast, boneless, frozen, seasoned, light and dark meat, roasted | 3 oz | 0.6 |
| Bagels, cinnamon-raisin | 3-1/2" bagel | 0.5 |
| Biscuits, plain or buttermilk, refrigerated dough, lower fat, baked | 2-1/4" biscuit | 0.5 |
| Bread, mixed-grain, toasted (includes whole-grain, 7-grain) | 1 slice | 0.5 |
| Bread, raisin, toasted, enriched | 1 slice | 0.5 |
| Cereals ready-to-eat, GENERAL MILLS, APPLE CINNAMON CHEERIOS | 3/4 cup | 0.5 |
| Cereals ready-to-eat, GENERAL MILLS, CHEERIOS | 1 cup | 0.5 |
| Cereals ready-to-eat, GENERAL MILLS, HONEY NUT CHEERIOS | 1 cup | 0.5 |
| Cereals ready-to-eat, GENERAL MILLS, WHEATIES | 1 cup | 0.5 |
| Cereals ready-to-eat, KELLOGG, KELLOGG'S Complete Wheat Bran Flakes | 3/4 cup | 0.5 |
| Cereals ready-to-eat, QUAKER, QUAKER OAT LIFE, plain | 3/4 cup | 0.5 |
| Cheese spread, pasteurized process, american, without | 1 oz | 0.5 |

| | | |
|---|---|---|
| di sodium phosphate | | |
| Cheese, cottage, lowfat, 2% milkfat | 1 cup | 0.5 |
| Cheese, feta | 1 oz | 0.5 |
| Cookies, vanilla sandwich with creme filling | 1 cookie | 0.5 |
| Corn, sweet, yellow, frozen, kernels cut off cob, boiled, drained, without salt | 1 cup | 0.5 |
| Cream, fluid, heavy whipping | 1 tbsp | 0.5 |
| Egg substitute, liquid | 1/4 cup | 0.5 |
| Eggnog | 1 cup | 0.5 |
| Macaroni and Cheese, canned entree | 1 cup | 0.5 |
| Milk, chocolate, fluid, commercial, reduced fat | 1 cup | 0.5 |
| Milk, chocolate, fluid, commercial, whole | 1 cup | 0.5 |
| Milk, reduced fat, fluid, 2% milkfat, with added vitamin A | 1 cup | 0.5 |
| Milk, whole, 3.25% milkfat | 1 cup | 0.5 |
| Onions, cooked, boiled, drained, without salt | 1 medium | 0.5 |
| Potatoes, baked, flesh, without salt | 1 potato | 0.5 |
| Raisins, seedless | 1 packet | 0.5 |
| Rutabagas, cooked, boiled, drained, without salt | 1 cup | 0.5 |
| Snacks, beef jerky, chopped and formed | 1 large piece | 0.5 |
| Snacks, pretzels, hard, plain, salted | 10 pretzels | 0.5 |
| Soup, chicken with rice, canned, prepared with equal volume water, commercial | 1 cup | 0.5 |

| | | |
|---|---|---|
| Soup, onion mix, dehydrated, dry form | 1 packet | 0.5 |
| Sour dressing, non-butterfat, cultured, filled cream-type | 1 tbsp | 0.5 |
| Yogurt, plain, low fat, 12 grams protein per 8 ounce | 8-oz container | 0.5 |
| Yogurt, plain, skim milk, 13 grams protein per 8 ounce | 8-oz container | 0.5 |
| Yogurt, plain, whole milk, 8 grams protein per 8 ounce | 8-oz container | 0.5 |
| Bread, egg | 1/2" slice | 0.4 |
| Bread, oatmeal | 1 slice | 0.4 |
| Bread, oatmeal, toasted | 1 slice | 0.4 |
| Bread, raisin, enriched | 1 slice | 0.4 |
| Bread, rye | 1 slice | 0.4 |
| Bread, wheat (includes wheat berry) | 1 slice | 0.4 |
| Bread, wheat, toasted (includes wheat berry) | 1 slice | 0.4 |
| Candies, milk chocolate coated raisins | 10 pieces | 0.4 |
| Catsup | 1 tbsp | 0.4 |
| Cereals ready-to-eat, GENERAL MILLS, BERRY BERRY KIX | 3/4 cup | 0.4 |
| Cereals ready-to-eat, GENERAL MILLS, HONEY NUT CLUSTERS | 1 cup | 0.4 |
| Cereals ready-to-eat, GENERAL MILLS, LUCKY CHARMS | 1 cup | 0.4 |
| Cereals ready-to-eat, GENERAL MILLS, Wheat CHEX | 1 cup | 0.4 |
| Cereals ready-to-eat, | 3/4 cup | 0.4 |

| | | |
|---|---|---|
| QUAKER, CAP'N CRUNCH | | |
| Cereals ready-to-eat, QUAKER, CAP'N CRUNCH with CRUNCHBERRIES | 3/4 cup | 0.4 |
| Cheese, cream | 1 tbsp | 0.4 |
| Cheese, mozzarella, part skim milk, low moisture | 1 oz | 0.4 |
| Cornmeal, degermed, enriched, yellow | 1 cup | 0.4 |
| Cornmeal, whole-grain, yellow | 1 cup | 0.4 |
| Cream substitute, liquid, with hydrogenated vegetable oil and soy protein | 1 tbsp | 0.4 |
| Cream, fluid, light whipping | 1 tbsp | 0.4 |
| Onions, raw | 1 whole | 0.4 |
| Pork and beef sausage, fresh, cooked | 2 links | 0.4 |
| Snacks,tortilla chips, nacho-flavor | 1 oz | 0.4 |
| Strawberries, raw | 1 strawberry | 0.4 |
| Syrups, chocolate, fudge-type | 1 tbsp | 0.4 |
| Wheat flour, white, all-purpose, enriched, bleached | 1 cup | 0.4 |
| Wheat flour, white, all-purpose, self-rising, enriched | 1 cup | 0.4 |
| Wheat flour, white, bread, enriched | 1 cup | 0.4 |
| Wheat flour, white, cake, enriched | 1 cup | 0.4 |
| Beets, canned, drained solids | 1 cup | 0.3 |
| Beets, cooked, boiled, | 1 cup | 0.3 |

| | | |
|---|---|---|
| drained | | |
| Bread, french or vienna (includes sourdough) | 1/2" slice | 0.3 |
| Bread, pumpernickel | 1 slice | 0.3 |
| Bread, pumpernickel, toasted | 1 slice | 0.3 |
| Bread, rye, toasted | 1 slice | 0.3 |
| Candies, fudge, chocolate, with nuts, prepared-from-recipe | 1 piece | 0.3 |
| Cereals ready-to-eat, GENERAL MILLS, GOLDEN GRAHAMS | 3/4 cup | 0.3 |
| Cereals ready-to-eat, GENERAL MILLS, REESE'S PUFFS | 3/4 cup | 0.3 |
| Cereals ready-to-eat, GENERAL MILLS, TRIX | 1 cup | 0.3 |
| Cereals ready-to-eat, KELLOGG, KELLOGG'S APPLE JACKS | 1 cup | 0.3 |
| Cereals ready-to-eat, KELLOGG, KELLOGG'S RICE KRISPIES TREATS Cereal | 3/4 cup | 0.3 |
| Cereals ready-to-eat, KELLOGG, KELLOGG'S SMACKS | 3/4 cup | 0.3 |
| Cereals ready-to-eat, QUAKER, CAP'N CRUNCH'S PEANUT BUTTER CRUNCH | 3/4 cup | 0.3 |
| Cereals ready-to-eat, wheat germ, toasted, plain | 1 tbsp | 0.3 |
| Cereals, CREAM OF WHEAT, regular, cooked | 1 cup | 0.3 |

| | | |
|---|---|---|
| with water, without salt | | |
| Chicken roll, light meat | 2 slices | 0.3 |
| Chicken, broilers or fryers, breast, meat only, cooked, roasted | 1/2 breast | 0.3 |
| Cocoa mix, powder | 3 heaping tsp | 0.3 |
| Corn, sweet, white, cooked, boiled, drained, without salt | 1 ear | 0.3 |
| Corn, sweet, yellow, cooked, boiled, drained, without salt | 1 ear | 0.3 |
| Corn, sweet, yellow, frozen, kernels on cob, cooked, boiled, drained, without salt | 1 ear | 0.3 |
| Cream, fluid, light (coffee cream or table cream) | 1 tbsp | 0.3 |
| Dessert topping, semi solid, frozen | 1 tbsp | 0.3 |
| Fish, salmon, pink, canned, solids with bone and liquid | 3 oz | 0.3 |
| Ice creams, vanilla, light | 1/2 cup | 0.3 |
| Milk, chocolate, fluid, commercial, lowfat | 1 cup | 0.3 |
| Mollusks, clam, mixed species, canned, drained solids | 3 oz | 0.3 |
| Nuts, coconut meat, dried (desiccated), sweetened, shredded | 1 cup | 0.3 |
| Oil, vegetable, corn, industrial and retail, all purpose salad or cooking | 1 tbsp | 0.3 |
| Olives, ripe, canned (small-extra large) | 5 large | 0.3 |
| Pineapple and grapefruit | 8 fl oz | 0.3 |

| | | |
|---|---|---|
| juice drink, canned | | |
| Pineapple and orange juice drink, canned | 8 fl oz | 0.3 |
| Rolls, hard (includes kaiser) | 1 roll | 0.3 |
| Salami, dry or hard, pork, beef | 2 slices | 0.3 |
| Sausage, Vienna, canned, chicken, beef, pork | 1 sausage | 0.3 |
| Strawberries, raw | 1 strawberry | 0.3 |
| Waterchestnuts, chinese, canned, solids and liquids | 1 cup | 0.3 |
| Watermelon, raw | 1 wedge | 0.3 |
| Bologna, beef and pork | 2 slices | 0.2 |
| Bread, italian | 1 slice | 0.2 |
| Candies, caramels | 1 piece | 0.2 |
| Candies, fudge, chocolate, prepared-from-recipe | 1 piece | 0.2 |
| Candies, M&M MARS, "M&M's" Milk Chocolate Candies | 10 pieces | 0.2 |
| Catsup | 1 packet | 0.2 |
| Cereals ready-to-eat, GENERAL MILLS, COCOA PUFFS | 1 cup | 0.2 |
| Cereals ready-to-eat, GENERAL MILLS, KIX | 1-1/3 cup | 0.2 |
| Cereals ready-to-eat, GENERAL MILLS, Whole Grain TOTAL | 3/4 cup | 0.2 |
| Cereals ready-to-eat, KELLOGG, KELLOGG'S PRODUCT 19 | 1 cup | 0.2 |
| Cereals ready-to-eat, KELLOGG, KELLOGG'S | 1 cup | 0.2 |

| SPECIAL K | | |
|---|---|---|
| Cheese, cottage, lowfat, 1% milkfat | 1 cup | 0.2 |
| Cheese, low fat, cheddar or colby | 1 oz | 0.2 |
| Cocoa mix, powder, prepared with water | 1 serving | 0.2 |
| Coffee, brewed from grounds, prepared with tap water | 6 fl oz | 0.2 |
| Cookies, vanilla wafers, lower fat | 1 cookie | 0.2 |
| Couscous, cooked | 1 cup | 0.2 |
| Crackers, melba toast, plain | 4 pieces | 0.2 |
| Cream substitute, powdered | 1 tsp | 0.2 |
| Cream, fluid, half and half | 1 tbsp | 0.2 |
| Dessert topping, pressurized | 1 tbsp | 0.2 |
| Egg, whole, cooked, hard-boiled | 1 large | 0.2 |
| Egg, whole, cooked, poached | 1 large | 0.2 |
| Egg, whole, raw, fresh | 1 extra large | 0.2 |
| Egg, whole, raw, fresh | 1 large | 0.2 |
| Fish, herring, Atlantic, pickled | 3 oz | 0.2 |
| Fish, tuna, light, canned in water, drained solids | 3 oz | 0.2 |
| Frozen yogurts, vanilla, soft-serve | 1/2 cup | 0.2 |
| Grapefruit juice, white, frozen concentrate, unsweetened, undiluted | 6-fl-oz can | 0.2 |
| Ice creams, chocolate | 1/2 cup | 0.2 |
| Ice creams, vanilla | 1/2 cup | 0.2 |

| | | |
|---|---|---|
| Jerusalem-artichokes, raw | 1 cup | 0.2 |
| Kohlrabi, cooked, boiled, drained, without salt | 1 cup | 0.2 |
| Lime juice, raw | juice of 1 lime | 0.2 |
| Malted drink mix, natural, with added nutrients, powder | 4-5 heaping tsp | 0.2 |
| Milk, buttermilk, fluid, cultured, lowfat | 1 cup | 0.2 |
| Milk, lowfat, fluid, 1% milkfat, with added vitamin A | 1 cup | 0.2 |
| Mollusks, clam, mixed species, raw | 3 oz | 0.2 |
| Mushrooms, canned, drained solids | 1 cup | 0.2 |
| Mushrooms, cooked, boiled, drained, without salt | 1 cup | 0.2 |
| Onions, dehydrated flakes | 1 tbsp | 0.2 |
| Orange juice, canned, unsweetened | 1 cup | 0.2 |
| Orange juice, frozen concentrate, unsweetened, diluted with 3 volume water | 1 cup | 0.2 |
| Orange juice, raw | 1 cup | 0.2 |
| Pears, canned, heavy syrup pack, solids and liquids | 1 half | 0.2 |
| Pears, canned, juice pack, solids and liquids | 1 half | 0.2 |
| Rice, white, long-grain, parboiled, enriched, dry | 1 cup | 0.2 |
| Rice, white, long-grain, regular, raw, enriched | 1 cup | 0.2 |
| Sandwich spread, pork, beef | 1 tbsp | 0.2 |
| Seaweed, spirulina, dried | 1 tbsp | 0.2 |

| | | |
|---|---|---|
| Snacks, rice cakes, brown rice, plain | 1 cake | 0.2 |
| Snacks, tortilla chips, plain, white corn | 1 oz | 0.2 |
| Soup, beef broth or bouillon, powder, dry | 1 packet | 0.2 |
| Soup, onion, dehydrated, prepared with water | 1 cup | 0.2 |
| Turnips, cooked, boiled, drained, without salt | 1 cup | 0.2 |
| Watermelon, raw | 1 cup | 0.2 |
| Yogurt, fruit, low fat, 10 grams protein per 8 ounce | 8-oz container | 0.2 |
| Alcoholic beverage, daiquiri, prepared-from-recipe | 2 fl oz | 0.1 |
| Alcoholic beverage, pina colada, prepared-from-recipe | 4.5 fl oz | 0.1 |
| Beets, cooked, boiled, drained | 1 beet | 0.1 |
| Bread, pita, white, enriched | 6-1/2" pita | 0.1 |
| Bread, pita, white, enriched | 4" pita | 0.1 |
| Bread, reduced-calorie, rye | 1 slice | 0.1 |
| Bread, reduced-calorie, white | 1 slice | 0.1 |
| Cake, angelfood, dry mix, prepared | 1 piece | 0.1 |
| Cake, sponge, commercially prepared | 1 shortcake | 0.1 |
| Candies, fudge, vanilla with nuts | 1 piece | 0.1 |
| Candies, fudge, vanilla, prepared-from-recipe | 1 piece | 0.1 |
| Candies, M&M MARS, STARBURST Fruit Chews | 1 piece | 0.1 |
| Candies, NESTLE, | 1 fun size | 0.1 |

| | | |
|---|---|---|
| BUTTERFINGER Bar | bar | |
| Cereals ready-to-eat, GENERAL MILLS, Corn CHEX | 1 cup | 0.1 |
| Cereals ready-to-eat, GENERAL MILLS, TOTAL Corn Flakes | 1-1/3 cup | 0.1 |
| Cereals ready-to-eat, KELLOGG, KELLOGG'S FROOT LOOPS | 1 cup | 0.1 |
| Cereals ready-to-eat, KELLOGG, KELLOGG'S FROSTED FLAKES | 3/4 cup | 0.1 |
| Cheese, parmesan, grated | 1 tbsp | 0.1 |
| Chocolate syrup | 1 tbsp | 0.1 |
| Cocoa mix, no sugar added, powder | 1/2 oz envelope | 0.1 |
| Cocoa, dry powder, unsweetened | 1 tbsp | 0.1 |
| Coffee, brewed, espresso, restaurant-prepared | 2 fl oz | 0.1 |
| Cookies, butter, commercially prepared, enriched | 1 cookie | 0.1 |
| Cookies, oatmeal, commercially prepared, fat-free | 1 cookie | 0.1 |
| Crackers, cheese, regular | 10 crackers | 0.1 |
| Crackers, matzo, plain | 1 matzo | 0.1 |
| Cream, sour, cultured | 1 tbsp | 0.1 |
| Cream, sour, reduced fat, cultured | 1 tbsp | 0.1 |
| Cream, whipped, cream topping, pressurized | 1 tbsp | 0.1 |

| | | |
|---|---|---|
| Crustaceans, crab, alaska king, imitation, made from surimi | 3 oz | 0.1 |
| Crustaceans, crab, blue, canned | 1 cup | 0.1 |
| Crustaceans, crab, blue, cooked, moist heat | 3 oz | 0.1 |
| Crustaceans, lobster, northern, cooked, moist heat | 3 oz | 0.1 |
| Dessert topping, powdered, 1.5 ounce prepared with 1/2 cup milk | 1 tbsp | 0.1 |
| Egg, whole, raw, fresh | 1 medium | 0.1 |
| Egg, yolk, raw, fresh | 1 large | 0.1 |
| Fish, cod, Atlantic, canned, solids and liquid | 3 oz | 0.1 |
| Fish, flatfish (flounder and sole species), cooked, dry heat | 1 fillet | 0.1 |
| Fish, flatfish (flounder and sole species), cooked, dry heat | 3 oz | 0.1 |
| Fish, pollock, walleye, cooked, dry heat | 1 fillet | 0.1 |
| Fish, pollock, walleye, cooked, dry heat | 3 oz | 0.1 |
| Fish, rockfish, Pacific, mixed species, cooked, dry heat | 1 fillet | 0.1 |
| Fish, rockfish, Pacific, mixed species, cooked, dry heat | 3 oz | 0.1 |
| Fish, salmon, chinook, smoked | 3 oz | 0.1 |
| Gravy, beef, canned | 1/4 cup | 0.1 |
| Gravy, chicken, canned | 1/4 cup | 0.1 |
| Horseradish, prepared | 1 tsp | 0.1 |

| | | |
|---|---|---|
| Jellies | 1 tbsp | 0.1 |
| Lime juice, canned or bottled, unsweetened | 1 tbsp | 0.1 |
| Mollusks, oyster, eastern, wild, raw | 6 medium | 0.1 |
| Mushrooms, shiitake, cooked, without salt | 1 cup | 0.1 |
| Mustard, prepared, yellow | 1 tsp or 1 packet | 0.1 |
| Nuts, coconut meat, raw | 1 piece | 0.1 |
| Oil, peanut, salad or cooking | 1 tbsp | 0.1 |
| Onions, raw | 1 slice | 0.1 |
| Orange juice, raw | juice from 1 orange | 0.1 |
| Peanut butter, chunk style, with salt | 1 tbsp | 0.1 |
| Peanut butter, smooth style, with salt | 1 tbsp | 0.1 |
| Pineapple, canned, heavy syrup pack, solids and liquids | 1 slice | 0.1 |
| Pineapple, canned, juice pack, solids and liquids | 1 slice | 0.1 |
| Pork Sausage, Fresh, Cooked | 1 patty | 0.1 |
| Pork Sausage, Fresh, Cooked | 2 links | 0.1 |
| Radishes, raw | 1 radish | 0.1 |
| Sauce, hoisin, ready-to-serve | 1 tbsp | 0.1 |
| Sauce, ready-to-serve, pepper or hot | 1 tsp | 0.1 |
| Snacks, popcorn, air-popped | 1 cup | 0.1 |
| Snacks, popcorn, cakes | 1 cake | 0.1 |
| Spices, onion powder | 1 tsp | 0.1 |

| | | |
|---|---|---|
| Alcoholic beverage, beer, light | 12 fl oz | 0.0 |
| Alcoholic beverage, beer, regular, all | 12 fl oz | 0.0 |
| Alcoholic beverage, distilled, all (gin, rum, vodka, whiskey) 80 proof | 1.5 fl oz | 0.0 |
| Alcoholic beverage, distilled, all (gin, rum, vodka, whiskey) 86 proof | 1.5 fl oz | 0.0 |
| Alcoholic beverage, distilled, all (gin, rum, vodka, whiskey) 90 proof | 1.5 fl oz | 0.0 |
| Alcoholic beverage, liqueur, coffee, 53 proof | 1.5 fl oz | 0.0 |
| Alcoholic beverage, wine, dessert, dry | 3.5 fl oz | 0.0 |
| Alcoholic beverage, wine, dessert, sweet | 3.5 fl oz | 0.0 |
| Apple juice, canned or bottled, unsweetened, without added ascorbic acid | 1 cup | 0.0 |
| Bamboo shoots, canned, drained solids | 1 cup | 0.0 |
| Beef, cured, dried | 1 oz | 0.0 |
| Beets, canned, drained solids | 1 beet | 0.0 |
| Bread, reduced-calorie, wheat | 1 slice | 0.0 |
| Cake, pound, commercially prepared, fat-free | 1 slice | 0.0 |
| Candies, gumdrops, starch jelly pieces | 10 bears | 0.0 |
| Candies, gumdrops, starch jelly pieces | 1 medium | 0.0 |

| | | |
|---|---|---|
| Candies, gumdrops, starch jelly pieces | 10 worms | 0.0 |
| Candies, hard | 1 small piece | 0.0 |
| Candies, hard | 1 piece | 0.0 |
| Candies, jellybeans | 10 large | 0.0 |
| Candies, marshmallows | 1 cup | 0.0 |
| Carambola, (starfruit), raw | 1 cup | 0.0 |
| Carambola, (starfruit), raw | 1 fruit | 0.0 |
| Carbonated beverage, club soda | 12 fl oz | 0.0 |
| Carbonated beverage, cola, contains caffeine | 12 fl oz | 0.0 |
| Carbonated beverage, ginger ale | 12 fl oz | 0.0 |
| Carbonated beverage, low calorie, cola or pepper-type, with aspartame, contains caffeine | 12 fl oz | 0.0 |
| Carbonated beverage, low calorie, other than cola or pepper, without caffeine | 12 fl oz | 0.0 |
| Carbonated beverage, root beer | 12 fl oz | 0.0 |
| Carbonated beverage, SPRITE, lemon-lime, without caffeine | 12 fl oz | 0.0 |
| Carob flour | 1 tbsp | 0.0 |
| Cereals ready-to-eat, GENERAL MILLS, Honey Nut CHEX | 3/4 cup | 0.0 |
| Cereals ready-to-eat, GENERAL MILLS, Rice CHEX | 1-1/4 cup | 0.0 |
| Cereals ready-to-eat, | 3/4 cup | 0.0 |

| | | |
|---|---|---|
| KELLOGG, KELLOGG'S COCOA KRISPIES | | |
| Cereals ready-to-eat, KELLOGG, KELLOGG'S Corn Flakes | 1 cup | 0.0 |
| Cereals ready-to-eat, KELLOGG, KELLOGG'S CORN POPS | 1 cup | 0.0 |
| Cereals ready-to-eat, KELLOGG, KELLOGG'S CRISPIX | 1 cup | 0.0 |
| Cereals ready-to-eat, KELLOGG, KELLOGG'S RICE KRISPIES | 1-1/4 cup | 0.0 |
| Cereals, corn grits, white, regular and quick, enriched, cooked with water, without salt | 1 cup | 0.0 |
| Cereals, corn grits, yellow, regular and quick, enriched, cooked with water, without salt | 1 cup | 0.0 |
| Cheese, cottage, nonfat, uncreamed, dry, large or small curd | 1 cup | 0.0 |
| Cheese, cream, fat free | 1 tbsp | 0.0 |
| Chicken, broilers or fryers, giblets, cooked, simmered | 1 cup | 0.0 |
| Chicken, liver, all classes, cooked, simmered | 1 liver | 0.0 |
| Coffee, instant, regular, prepared with water | 6 fl oz | 0.0 |
| Cookies, brownies, dry mix, special dietary, prepared | 1 brownie | 0.0 |
| Corn, sweet, yellow, canned, cream style, regular pack | 1 cup | 0.0 |

| | | |
|---|---|---|
| Corn, sweet, yellow, canned, vacuum pack, regular pack | 1 cup | 0.0 |
| Cornstarch | 1 tbsp | 0.0 |
| Crustaceans, shrimp, mixed species, canned | 3 oz | 0.0 |
| Egg, white, raw, fresh | 1 large | 0.0 |
| Frankfurter, chicken | 1 frank | 0.0 |
| Frozen novelties, ice type, pop | 1 bar (2 fl oz) | 0.0 |
| Fruit butters, apple | 1 tbsp | 0.0 |
| Fruit punch drink, with added nutrients, canned | 8 fl oz | 0.0 |
| Garlic, raw | 1 clove | 0.0 |
| Gelatin desserts, dry mix, prepared with water | 1/2 cup | 0.0 |
| Gelatin desserts, dry mix, reduced calorie, with aspartame, prepared with water | 1/2 cup | 0.0 |
| Grape drink, canned | 8 fl oz | 0.0 |
| Grapefruit juice, white, canned, sweetened | 1 cup | 0.0 |
| Grapefruit juice, white, canned, unsweetened | 1 cup | 0.0 |
| Grapefruit juice, white, frozen concentrate, unsweetened, diluted with 3 volume water | 1 cup | 0.0 |
| Grapefruit juice, white, raw | 1 cup | 0.0 |
| Grapefruit, raw, pink and red, all areas | 1/2 grapefruit | 0.0 |
| Grapefruit, raw, white, all areas | 1/2 grapefruit | 0.0 |
| Grapefruit, sections, canned, light syrup pack, solids and | 1 cup | 0.0 |

Vitamin K Levels in Common Foods

| liquids | | |
|---|---|---|
| Gravy, turkey, canned | 1/4 cup | 0.0 |
| Ham, chopped, not canned | 2 slices | 0.0 |
| Ham, sliced, extra lean | 2 slices | 0.0 |
| Ham, sliced, regular (approximately 11% fat) | 2 slices | 0.0 |
| Honey | 1 tbsp | 0.0 |
| Jams and preserves | 1 tbsp | 0.0 |
| Lard | 1 tbsp | 0.0 |
| Leavening agents, baking powder, double-acting, sodium aluminum sulfate | 1 tsp | 0.0 |
| Leavening agents, baking powder, double-acting, straight phosphate | 1 tsp | 0.0 |
| Leavening agents, baking powder, low-sodium | 1 tsp | 0.0 |
| Leavening agents, baking soda | 1 tsp | 0.0 |
| Leavening agents, cream of tartar | 1 tsp | 0.0 |
| Leavening agents, yeast, baker's, active dry | 1 tsp | 0.0 |
| Leavening agents, yeast, baker's, active dry | 1 pkg | 0.0 |
| Leavening agents, yeast, baker's, compressed | 1 cake | 0.0 |
| Lemon juice, canned or bottled | 1 cup | 0.0 |
| Lemon juice, canned or bottled | 1 tbsp | 0.0 |
| Lemon juice, raw | juice of 1 lemon | 0.0 |
| Lemonade, frozen concentrate, white, prepared | 8 fl oz | 0.0 |

| | | |
|---|---|---|
| with water | | |
| Lemonade, low calorie, with aspartame, powder, prepared with water | 8 fl oz | 0.0 |
| Lemons, raw, without peel | 1 lemon | 0.0 |
| Macaroni, cooked, enriched | 1 cup | 0.0 |
| Milk, buttermilk, dried | 1 tbsp | 0.0 |
| Milk, canned, evaporated, nonfat | 1 cup | 0.0 |
| Milk, dry, nonfat, instant, with added vitamin A | 1/3 cup | 0.0 |
| Milk, nonfat, fluid, with added vitamin A (fat free or skim) | 1 cup | 0.0 |
| Mushrooms, raw | 1 cup | 0.0 |
| Mushrooms, shiitake, dried | 1 mushroom | 0.0 |
| Noodles, egg, cooked, enriched | 1 cup | 0.0 |
| Nuts, almonds | 1 oz (24 nuts) | 0.0 |
| Nuts, brazilnuts, dried, unblanched | 1 oz (6-8 nuts) | 0.0 |
| Nuts, macadamia nuts, dry roasted, with salt added | 1 oz (10-12 nuts) | 0.0 |
| Oranges, raw, all commercial varieties | 1 cup | 0.0 |
| Oranges, raw, all commercial varieties | 1 orange | 0.0 |
| Peanuts, all types, dry-roasted, with salt | 1 oz (approx 28) | 0.0 |
| Peanuts, all types, dry-roasted, without salt | 1 oz (approx 28) | 0.0 |
| Peanuts, all types, oil- | 1 oz | 0.0 |

| | | |
|---|---|---|
| roasted, with salt | | |
| Pie fillings, apple, canned | 1/8 of 21 oz can | 0.0 |
| Pork, cured, bacon, cooked, broiled, pan-fried or roasted | 3 medium slices | 0.0 |
| Pork, cured, canadian-style bacon, grilled | 2 slices | 0.0 |
| Pork, cured, ham, extra lean and regular, canned, roasted | 3 oz | 0.0 |
| Pork, cured, ham, whole, separable lean and fat, roasted | 3 oz | 0.0 |
| Pork, cured, ham, whole, separable lean only, roasted | 3 oz | 0.0 |
| Pork, fresh, leg (ham), whole, separable lean and fat, cooked, roasted | 3 oz | 0.0 |
| Pork, fresh, leg (ham), whole, separable lean only, cooked, roasted | 3 oz | 0.0 |
| Pork, fresh, loin, center loin (chops), bone-in, separable lean and fat, cooked, pan-fried | 3 oz | 0.0 |
| Pork, fresh, loin, center loin (chops), bone-in, separable lean only, cooked, pan-fried | 3 oz | 0.0 |
| Pork, fresh, shoulder, arm picnic, separable lean and fat, cooked, braised | 3 oz | 0.0 |
| Pork, fresh, shoulder, arm picnic, separable lean only, cooked, braised | 3 oz | 0.0 |
| Pork, fresh, spareribs, separable lean and fat, cooked, braised | 3 oz | 0.0 |

| | | |
|---|---|---|
| Puddings, vanilla, ready-to-eat | 4 oz | 0.0 |
| Rice, white, long-grain, parboiled, enriched, cooked | 1 cup | 0.0 |
| Rice, white, long-grain, precooked or instant, enriched, prepared | 1 cup | 0.0 |
| Rice, white, long-grain, regular, cooked | 1 cup | 0.0 |
| Salt, table | 1 tsp | 0.0 |
| Sauce, barbecue sauce | 1 tbsp | 0.0 |
| Sauce, teriyaki, ready-to-serve | 1 tbsp | 0.0 |
| Seeds, sesame butter, tahini, from roasted and toasted kernels (most common type) | 1 tbsp | 0.0 |
| Seeds, sesame seed kernels, dried (decorticated) | 1 tbsp | 0.0 |
| Sherbet, orange | 1/2 cup | 0.0 |
| Snacks, pork skins, plain | 1 oz | 0.0 |
| Soup, chicken noodle, canned, prepared with equal volume water, commercial | 1 cup | 0.0 |
| Soup, stock, fish, home-prepared | 1 cup | 0.0 |
| Soy sauce made from soy and wheat (shoyu) | 1 tbsp | 0.0 |
| Spaghetti, cooked, enriched, without added salt | 1 cup | 0.0 |
| Spices, celery seed | 1 tsp | 0.0 |
| Spices, garlic powder | 1 tsp | 0.0 |
| Sugars, brown | 1 tsp | 0.0 |
| Sugars, granulated | 1 tsp | 0.0 |
| Sugars, powdered | 1 tbsp | 0.0 |

| | | |
|---|---|---|
| Syrups, corn, light | 1 tbsp | 0.0 |
| Syrups, maple | 1 tbsp | 0.0 |
| Syrups, table blends, pancake | 1 tbsp | 0.0 |
| Syrups, table blends, pancake, reduced-calorie | 1 tbsp | 0.0 |
| Tangerine juice, canned, sweetened | 1 cup | 0.0 |
| Tangerines, (mandarin oranges), canned, light syrup pack | 1 cup | 0.0 |
| Tangerines, (mandarin oranges), raw | 1 tangerine | 0.0 |
| Tapioca, pearl, dry | 1 cup | 0.0 |
| Tea, brewed, prepared with tap water | 6 fl oz | 0.0 |
| Tea, herb, chamomile, brewed | 6 fl oz | 0.0 |
| Tea, herb, other than chamomile, brewed | 6 fl oz | 0.0 |
| Tea, instant, sweetened with sodium saccharin, lemon-flavored, prepared | 8 fl oz | 0.0 |
| Tea, instant, sweetened with sugar, lemon-flavored, without added ascorbic acid, powder, prepared | 8 fl oz | 0.0 |
| Tea, instant, unsweetened, powder, prepared | 8 fl oz | 0.0 |
| Tortillas, ready-to-bake or -fry, corn | 1 tortilla | 0.0 |
| Turkey, all classes, light meat, cooked, roasted | 3 oz | 0.0 |
| Vanilla extract | 1 tsp | 0.0 |
| Vinegar, cider | 1 tbsp | 0.0 |

| Water, municipal | 8 fl oz | 0.0 |

# ABOUT THE AUTHOR

**Timothy S. Harlan, M.D.,** is a practicing, board-certified Internist and is currently the Medical Director of Outpatient Clinics, Associate Chief of General Internal Medicine, and Assistant Clinical Professor of Medicine at the Tulane University School of Medicine in New Orleans, Louisiana. Dr. Harlan attended medical school at the Emory University School of Medicine, Atlanta, GA and pursued his residency at Emory University School of Medicine Affiliated Hospitals in Atlanta, GA.

Visit his web site at www.DrGourmet.com to find hundreds of Coumadin-safe recipes.

Made in the USA
Coppell, TX
05 November 2022

85783757R10068